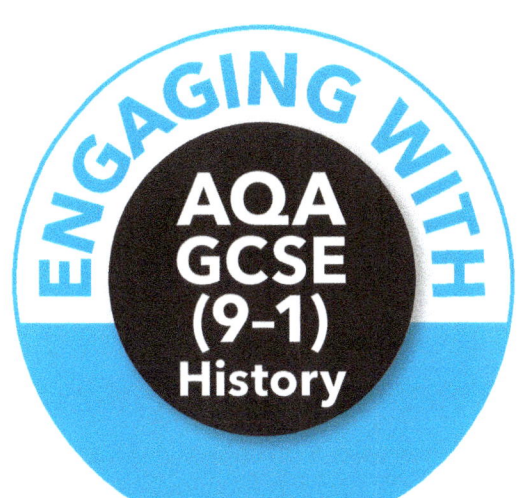

HEALTH & THE PEOPLE c1000 TO THE PRESENT DAY

THEMATIC STUDY

DALE BANHAM
IAN DAWSON

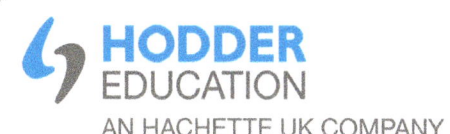

The Publishers would like to thank the following for permission to reproduce copyright material.

Photo credits

p.8t © Wellcome Collection, London/http://creativecommons.org/licenses/by/4.0/; **p.8tm** © imageBROKER / Alamy Stock Photo; **p.8bm** © Wellcome Collection, London/http://creativecommons.org/licenses/by/4.0/; **p.8b** Ms 146/1513 The tears and the suffering of Death, written by Jean Charlier de Gerson (1363–1429) (vellum), French School, (15th century) / Musee Conde, Chantilly, France / © MEPL / Bridgeman Images; **p.12** © Science History Images/Alamy Stock Photo; **p.15tl** © Gianni Dagli Orti/REX/Shutterstock; **p.15tr** © Granger Historical Picture Archive/Alamy Stock Photo; **p.15b** Ms 146/1513 The tears and the suffering of Death, written by Jean Charlier de Gerson (1363–1429) (vellum), French School, (15th century) / Musee Conde, Chantilly, France / © MEPL / Bridgeman Images; **p.16** © Gianni Dagli Orti/REX/Shutterstock; **p.19** © Photo The Morgan Library & Museum / Art Resource, NY/Scala, Florence; **p.22** © Gianni Dagli Orti/REX/Shutterstock; **p.24** The Black Death (gouache on paper), Nicolle, Pat (Patrick) (1907–95) / Private Collection / © Look and Learn / Bridgeman Images; **p.25** © The Print Collector / Alamy Stock Photo; **p.27** © The Print Collector / Alamy Stock Photo; **p.30** © The Granger Collection / Alamy Stock Photo; **p.32** Wellcome Collection, London/http://creativecommons.org/licenses/by/4.0/; **p.33** Wellcome Collection.https://creativecommons.org/licenses/by/4.0/; **p.34** Wellcome Collection.https://creativecommons.org/licenses/by/4.0/; **p.36l** © Wellcome Collection, London/http://creativecommons.org/licenses/by/4.0/; **p.36r** Wellcome Collection.https://creativecommons.org/licenses/by/4.0/; **p.37** © Cci/REX/Shutterstock; **p.38** © Wellcome Collection, London/http://creativecommons.org/licenses/by/4.0/; **p.39** © Wellcome Collection, London/http://creativecommons.org/licenses/by/4.0/; **p.40** © Wellcome Collection, London/http://creativecommons.org/licenses/by/4.0/; **p.41** © Granger Historical Picture Archive / Alamy Stock Photo; **p.45tr** © Wellcome Collection, London/http://creativecommons.org/licenses/by/4.0/; **p.45bl** © Wellcome Collection, London/http://creativecommons.org/licenses/by/4.0/; **p.48** © Wellcome Collection, London/http://creativecommons.org/licenses/by/4.0/; **p.50** Wellcome Collection.https://creativecommons.org/licenses/by/4.0; **p.52** © Hulton Archive/Getty Images; **p.53** Wellcome Collection.https://creativecommons.org/licenses/by/4.0; **p.55t** Science Museum, London. https://creativecommons.org/licenses/by/4.0; **p.55b** Wellcome Collection.https://creativecommons.org/licenses/by/4.0; **p.56** © Wellcome Collection, London/http://creativecommons.org/licenses/by/4.0/; **p.58** © Wellcome Collection, London/http://creativecommons.org/licenses/by/4.0/; **p.59** © Chronicle / Alamy Stock Photo; **p.63** © Wellcome Collection, London/http://creativecommons.org/licenses/by/4.0/; **p.64** © World History Archive / Alamy Stock Photo; **p.65** Wellcome Collection. https://creativecommons.org/licenses/by/4.0/; **p.67** © Elizabeth Leyden/Alamy Stock Photo; **p.69t** World History Archive/Alamy Stock Photo; **p.69b** Bettman/Getty Images; **p.71** © Chronicle / Alamy Stock Photo; **p.72** Keystone Press/Alamy Stock Photo; **p.74** © Hulton-Deutsch Collection/CORBIS/Corbis via Getty Images; **p.76** A. BARRINGTON BROWN, © GONVILLE & CAIUS COLLEGE/COLOURED BY SCIENCE PHOTO LIBRARY; **p.77** © Jonty Clark; **p.79** © SSPL/Getty Images; **p.80** © Hi-Story/Alamy Stock Photo; **p.81** © EPSTOCK - Fotolia; **p.85** Library of Congress Prints and Photographs Division Washington, D.C., LC-B2- 578-7; **p.87** Cartoon by Leslie Gilbert Illingworth, 'Here's to the brave new world!', Daily Mail; 2/12/1942 © Daily Mail; **p.89** © Punch Cartoon Library / TopFoto; **p.93** Source: Cancer Research UK, accessed March 2019

Note: The wording and sentence structure of some written sources have been adapted and simplified to make them accessible to all pupils while faithfully preserving the sense of the originals.

Every effort has been made to trace all copyright holders, but if any have been inadvertently overlooked, the Publishers will be pleased to make the necessary arrangements at the first opportunity.

Although every effort has been made to ensure that website addresses are correct at time of going to press, Hodder Education cannot be held responsible for the content of any website mentioned in this book. It is sometimes possible to find a relocated web page by typing in the address of the home page for a website in the URL window of your browser.

Hachette UK's policy is to use papers that are natural, renewable and recyclable products and made from wood in grown well-managed forests and other controlled sources. The logging and manufacturing processes are expected to conform to the environmental regulations of the country of origin.

Orders: please contact Hachette UK Distribution, Hely Hutchinson Centre, Milton Road, Didcot, Oxfordshire, OX11 7HH. Telephone: +44 (0)1235 827827. Email education@hachette.co.uk. Lines are open from 9 a.m. to 5 p.m., Monday to Friday. You can also order through our website: www.hoddereducation.co.uk

ISBN: 978 1 5104 5892 5

© Dale Banham and Ian Dawson 2019

First published in 2019 by

Hodder Education

An Hachette UK Company

Carmelite House

50 Victoria Embankment

London EC4Y 0DZ

www.hoddereducation.co.uk

Impression number   7

Year   2024

All rights reserved. Apart from any use permitted under UK copyright law, no part of this publication may be reproduced or transmitted in any form or by any means, electronic or mechanical, including photocopying and recording, or held within any information storage and retrieval system, without permission in writing from the publisher or under licence from the Copyright Licensing Agency Limited. Further details of such licences (for reprographic reproduction) may be obtained from the Copyright Licensing Agency Limited, www.cla.co.uk

Cover photo 'An ill man who is being bled by his doctor.' Coloured etching by J. Sneyd, 1804, after J. Gillray James Gillray. Wellcome Collection. CC BY.

Illustrations by Peter Lubach, D'AVILA Illustration Agency and Aptara

Typeset in India by Aptara

Printed in the UK

A catalogue record for this title is available from the British Library.

CONTENTS

Introduction to the Thematic Study

Part 1: The Middle Ages, c1000–1500: Medicine stands still

Period introduction: The Middle Ages 12
1.1 Introducing ... Claudius Galen 12

1 Medieval medicine 14
1.2 Beliefs about the causes of illness and methods of prevention and treatment in the Middle Ages 14
1.3 The medieval doctor 16

2 Medical progress in the Middle Ages 18
2.1 The contribution of Christianity to medical progress and treatment 18
2.2 The nature and importance of Islamic medicine 20
2.3 Surgery in medieval times 22

3 Public health in the Middle Ages 24
3.1 Towns and monasteries 24
3.2 Case study: The Black Death in Britain 26
3.3 Middle Ages period review 28

Part 2: Renaissance Britain, c1500–1800: The beginnings of change

Period introduction: The Renaissance period, c1500–1800 30
4.1 Introducing ... Andreas Vesalius 30

4 The impact of the Renaissance on Britain 32
4.2 How knowledge of anatomy improved 32
4.3 The work of William Harvey 34
4.4 The work of Ambroise Paré 36

5 Dealing with disease 38
5.1 Traditional and new methods of treating illness 38
5.2 Case study: The Great Plague of 1665 40
5.3 The growth of hospitals 42
5.4 Changes to the training and status of surgeons and physicians 44

6 Prevention of disease 46
6.1 Edward Jenner and the smallpox vaccination 46
6.2 Renaissance period review 48

Part 3: The nineteenth century, c1800–1900: A revolution in medicine

Period introduction: The nineteenth century 50
7.1 Introducing ... Louis Pasteur 50

7 The development of the Germ Theory and its impact on the treatment of disease in Britain 52
7.2 Robert Koch and microbe hunting 52
7.3 Vaccinations, magic bullets and everyday treatments 54

8 A revolution in surgery 56
8.1 The problems facing surgeons in the early 1800s 56
8.2 James Simpson and chloroform 58
8.3 Antiseptics: Lister and carbolic acid 60
8.4 Aseptic surgery and better surgical procedures 62

9 Improvements in public health 64
9.1 Public health problems in industrial Britain 64
9.2 The factors behind public health improvement: Part 1 66
9.3 The factors behind public health improvement: Part 2 68
9.4 Nineteenth century period review 70

Part 4: The twentieth century, c1900–today: Modern medicine

Period introduction: The twentieth century 72
10.1 Introducing ... Alexander Fleming – and the discovery of penicillin 72

10 Modern treatment of disease 74
10.2 The development of penicillin 74
10.3 The development of the pharmaceutical industry, new treatments and new diseases 76

11 The impact of war and technology on surgery 78
11.1 The impact of the First and Second World Wars on surgery 78
11.2 Modern surgical methods 80
11.3 The factors behind improvements in surgery 82

12 Modern public health 84
12.1 The Liberal social reforms 84
12.2 The impact of two world wars on public health, poverty and housing 86
12.3 The creation and development of the National Health Service 88
12.4 Costs, choices and the issues of healthcare in the twenty-first century 90
12.5 Twentieth century period review 92

Glossary 94

Index 96

0.1 Your exam: What is assessed and how

The GCSE course that you are following is made up of four different studies.

	Paper 1: Understanding the modern world	Paper 2: Shaping the nation
What is assessed?	**Section A: Period study** This focuses on key developments in a country's history over at least a 50-year period	**Section A: Thematic study** This looks at key developments in Britain over a long period of time (at least 800 years)
	Section B: Wider world depth study This focuses on international conflict and tension over a period of 20–25 years	**Section B: British depth study including the historic environment** This focuses on a period of British history over a short period of time (under 40 years) and includes the study of a specific historic environment
How is it assessed?	Written exam: 2 hours 50% of your GCSE (84 marks) Section A – 6 compulsory questions (40 marks) Section B – 4 compulsory questions (40 marks plus 4 marks for spelling, punctuation and grammar)	Written exam: 2 hours 50% of your GCSE (84 marks) **Section A – 4 compulsory questions (40 marks)** Section B – 4 compulsory questions (40 marks plus 4 marks for spelling, punctuation and grammar)

This book prepares you for the Thematic Study, **Britain: Health and the People, c1000 to the present day**.

It focuses on how medicine and health developed in Britain over a long period of time. You will study:

- how developments in medicine and public health related to the **key features and characteristics of the periods** in which they took place
- how the **pace and scale** of medical development has varied at different times
- the **causes and consequences** of the developments that took place
- the **significance** of key developments, individuals and events.

Period and theme	Key content (topics)	Period review pages
Part 1: The Middle Ages, c1000–1500 *Medicine stands still*	• Medieval medicine • Medical progress (in hospitals and surgery) • Public health in the Middle Ages	Pages 28–29
Part 2: Renaissance Britain, c1500–1800 *The beginnings of change*	• The impact of the Renaissance on Britain • Dealing with disease • Prevention of disease	Pages 48–49
Part 3: The nineteenth century, c1800–1900 *A revolution in medicine*	• The impact of the Germ Theory on the treatment of disease in Britain • A revolution in surgery • Improvements in public health	Pages 70–71
Part 4: The twentieth century, c1900–today *Modern medicine*	• Modern treatment of disease • The impact of war and technology on surgery • Modern public health	Pages 92–93

> **Revision Tip**
>
> **Break down your revision into manageable chunks of content**
>
> This book is organised into the four parts and the twelve topics of the specification. At the end of each topic, make sure you review and revise what you have just covered. The 'Exam Practice', 'Recall Challenge' and 'Review' features will help you do this.

How the Thematic Study will be examined

You will be examined on your knowledge and understanding of the Thematic Study in Paper 2. You will apply your knowledge and understanding to:

- explaining and analysing second-order historical concepts, such as continuity, change, cause, consequence, significance, similarity and difference
- analysing and evaluating historical sources (contemporary to the period).

The table below shows the types of questions you will be asked.

This book will give you step-by-step guidance on how to tackle each type of question.

	Type of question	Guidance	Marks	Timing	Advice and practice
1	How useful is Source …	The source could be visual or written. It will relate to a key event, development or individual. Focus on **why** the source is useful. Use the content of the source, the provenance of the source and your contextual knowledge to evaluate the usefulness of the source.	8	10 minutes	Pages 33, 63, 71, 89, 93
2	Explain the significance of …	Think then **and** now. What was the importance of a key event, individual or development at the time? (short-term impact) AND … What was the importance over time? (long-term consequences, influence today)	8	10 minutes	Pages 35, 63, 71, 83, 93
3	Explain two ways in which they are similar/different?	Focus on the question – focus on similarities **or** differences; you do not need to do both. Identify and explain two ways in which the two events are similar/different. Think: • Are the reasons why the two events happened similar/different? • Are there similarities/differences in how the events developed or how people responded to them? • Are there similarities/differences in the impacts, outcomes or results of the events?	8	10 minutes	Pages 43, 71, 83, 93
4	Evaluate factors	This is an essay question, requiring you to reach a **judgement**. Aim to evaluate the factor stated in the question first. Weigh how important it was compared to two other factors. Reach a judgement – was it the most important factor? Use your knowledge of all four parts of the specification to support your argument.	20 (16 + 4 for SPaG)	25 minutes	Pages 83, 93

Revision Tips

Make exam practice part of your revision

Exam Tips give you step-by-step guidance on how to tackle each type of question. Effective revision is not just learning the content. You need to understand what each type of question in the exam is asking you to think about and to practise delivering it.

Take responsibility

Reflect on your strengths and weaknesses. What question types do you struggle with? Spend more time practising the types of questions you find most difficult. Use feedback from your teacher to improve your approach.

0.2 The Big Picture: Identify the key questions

> **Reflect**
>
> The period summaries below identify people and events that have shaped the people's health in Britain over the last 1000 years. They also show the big questions you will cover. However, top history students do not only answer other people's questions, they also ask questions of their own! As you read each summary, note down your own questions (large or small) about each period.

PART 1: The Middle Ages, c1000–1500: *Medicine stands still*

Big question: Why did medicine and public health change so little during the Middles Ages?

Ideas about the causes of disease and illness

- Some medieval people believed God sent illness to punish people for their sins. Others believed that people who became ill had breathed in bad air.
- Specialist doctors called **physicians** treated the rich.
- In the 1200s, universities were set up and physicians were trained there. They read the works of **Galen** (a doctor from Ancient Rome) and Arab doctors such as Ibn Sina.
- Galen blamed sickness on the four **humours** (liquids) in the body being out of balance.

Methods of prevention and treatment

- Most medieval people would pray to God for forgiveness and healing.
- If a sick person went to a physician, he checked their urine to see if their humours were out of balance. He balanced them by **bleeding** (taking blood from the body) or purging (making the person vomit).
- Most people could not afford to see a physician. They were treated at home or by the local wise woman with **herbal remedies**.
- There were hospitals but they provided prayer, rest and food, not medical treatments.
- When a terribly bad outbreak of **plague** called the **Black Death** arrived in 1348, it killed around 40 per cent of the population. People could not treat those who had the disease or stop the plague spreading.

PART 2: Renaissance Britain, c1500–1800: *The beginnings of change*

Big question: How far were the ideas of Hippocrates and Galen challenged during the Renaissance?

Ideas about the causes of disease and illness

- Most people continued to believe that God or bad air or unbalanced humours made people sick.
- **Andreas Vesalius** improved knowledge of **anatomy** (the structure of the body) by dissecting dead bodies.
- **William Harvey** discovered that blood circulates round the body.
- Knowledge spread more quickly because of the invention of the printing press.

Methods of prevention and treatment

- Vesalius and Harvey improved medical knowledge, but they did not cure illnesses. Prayer and herbal remedies remained common treatments. Physicians still used bleeding and purging to balance humours.
- **Ambroise Paré** improved surgery and designed artificial limbs.
- **Barber-surgeons** carried out simple operations outside of the body but internal surgery was impossible without **anaesthetics**.
- There were more hospitals and they started to provide specialised care (for example, maternity wards).
- There was a serious outbreak of plague in London in 1665 but, just like in 1348, no one could stop it.
- In the 1700s, there was growing interest in scientific medicine and old ideas were challenged. New methods of treatment were tried out, for example, **Edward Jenner** invented **vaccination** to prevent people catching smallpox.

PART 3: The nineteenth century, c1800–1900: *A revolution in medicine*

Big question: How did the Germ Theory revolutionise medicine and public health?

Ideas about the causes of disease and illness

- In 1861, **Louis Pasteur** published his **Germ Theory** which showed that bacteria (**germs**) cause diseases. He carried out experiments to prove his theory was correct.
- However, some people still believed that bad air caused illness because diseases spread most rapidly in the dirtiest, smelliest industrial towns.

Methods of prevention and treatment

- Pasteur's theory led to treatments for killer diseases.
- Germ Theory also led to the development of **antiseptics** to prevent infection during surgery and helped persuade governments to pass laws to improve **public health**.
- Surgery was also improved by better scientific knowledge (particularly in chemistry) and the development of anaesthetics that prevented patients from experiencing pain during operations.
- Meanwhile, improvements in engineering helped to provide the sewer systems that would clean up the growing towns and cities during the Industrial Revolution.
- Not everything changed. People still used herbal remedies, some of which did help sick people. People still had to pay to see a doctor and nearly one in five babies died before their first birthday.
- However, **life expectancy** was beginning to rise. By 1900, people on average had a life expectancy nearer to 50 than 40 (which had been the case for centuries).

PART 4: The twentieth century, c1900 to today: *Modern medicine*

Big question: Why has life expectancy increased so dramatically in the last 100 years?

Ideas about the causes of disease and illness

- In the 1950s, scientists discovered the existence of **DNA**, the 'building blocks' of the human body. This led to much more research which identified the individual **genes** that cause some illnesses.

Methods of prevention and treatment

- Developments in science and technology greatly improved surgery, for example by identifying blood groups which made blood **transfusions** effective.
- The discovery and development of chemical drugs and then **antibiotics** in the 1940s saved millions of lives by providing cures for illnesses and infections.
- Wars forced governments to invest more in improving public health. During the twentieth century, governments introduced better education, housing and public health provision.
- In 1942, the **Beveridge Report** (produced by **William Beveridge**) created the plan for the National Health Service (**NHS**), which began in 1948. For the first time, the NHS provided everyone with free treatment from a doctor, so they were more likely to get help before an illness became serious.
- The result of all of these developments is that people born today will, on average, live at least twice as long as people born in 1800.

0.3 Factors that help to explain change and continuity in medicine

Research & Record

What factors influenced the history of medicine?

We are incredibly lucky to be living now and not 500 or even 100 years ago. As Graph 1 shows, we live far longer than our ancestors. We are healthier and have a greater chance of surviving major illnesses.

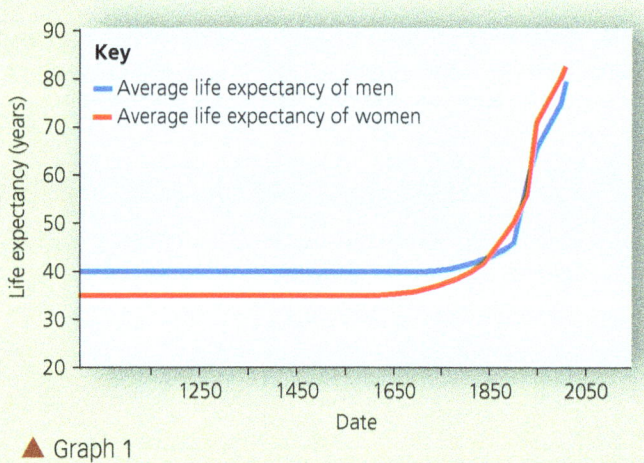
▲ Graph 1

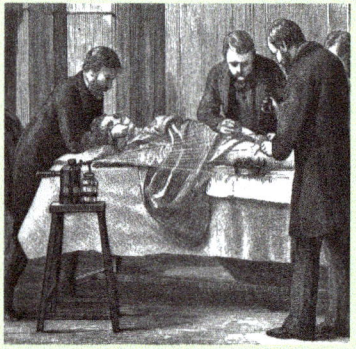
▲ Picture A

So why has medicine changed so much in recent times? That's what this course is all about. The cards on page 9 show the main factors that have affected medicine and health.

1. Pictures A–D show people being treated during different periods. Which time period does each image show?
2. Can you match one factor from page 9 to each picture?
3. Look back at the Big Picture on pages 6–7. What factors can you see influencing medicine and health in each period?
4. Make a large copy of a table like this to record your research. Keep this table and add to it throughout your course. Make sure you provide evidence to support your answers.

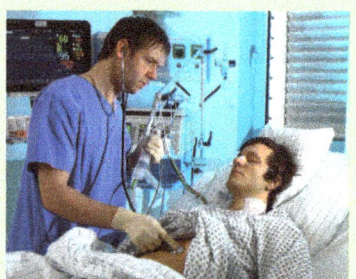
▲ Picture B

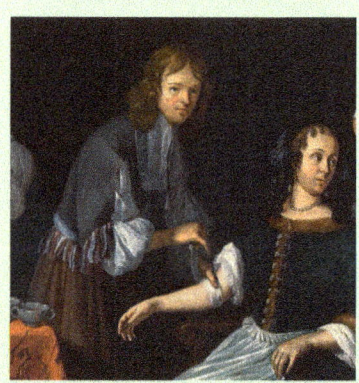
▲ Picture C

Period	Factors that influenced developments	Evidence
Medicine stands still (c1000–1500)	Religion	Hospitals were set up and run by the Church.
The beginnings of change (c1500–1800)		
A revolution in medicine (c1800–1900)		
Modern medicine (c1900–today)		

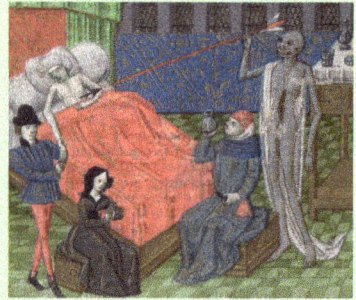
▲ Picture D

Beliefs – superstition and religion

Religious beliefs have both encouraged and inhibited change. For example, in the medieval period, both the Christian and Islamic religions set up hospitals and encouraged people to care for sick people. However, in medieval Britain, the Christian Church also discouraged people from challenging old ideas and developing new ones.

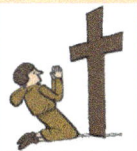

The role of individuals

Individuals have greatly influenced medicine and public health. For example, during the Renaissance, individuals such as Vesalius and Harvey increased knowledge of how the body is structured (anatomy) and the way that it works (**physiology**).

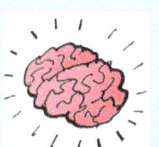

Communication

Throughout history, books have helped to spread medical ideas. During the medieval period, doctors in Britain were most influenced by books written by Galen and Islamic doctors. The invention of the printing press during the Renaissance period enabled books to be produced far more accurately and quickly.

Chance

Sometimes, new discoveries are made by chance. For example, during the Renaissance period, Paré tried a new technique for treating gunshot wounds only because he happened to run out of boiling oil.

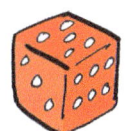

War

New surgical techniques can be tried out during wartime because there are so many serious injuries to treat. War led to the development of plastic surgery. After the First World War, surgeons needed to reconstruct the faces of soldiers who had been disfigured by explosives.

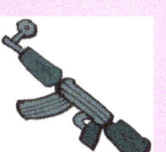

Government

In modern medicine, government plays a crucial role. During the nineteenth century, it passed laws to force local town councils to provide clean water for people. Since the creation of the NHS in the 1940s, the government uses a large part of the taxes it collects to fund the service and to pay for medical research and vaccination programmes.

Science and technology

Developments in science and technological improvements have transformed medicine in the last 200 years. New inventions and equipment, such as x-ray machines, body scanners and lasers, have revolutionised the way that illness is diagnosed and treated.

Revision Tip

Take responsibility

Question 4 in the exam will test your knowledge and understanding of these key factors and the role they played in each period of medicine. This question carries the most marks and the more care you give to completing this table, the better able you will be to write a good answer.

0.4 Key features: How this book works

The tasks in this book will help you learn what you need to know and how to apply your knowledge to answer exam questions effectively. They are your '**Steps to success**'.

Research & Record

Gets the **learning** into your head in the first place and into your notebook. Starts you thinking in a way that will help you produce good answers to the exam questions.

Each **research question** reflects an issue that the examiners will expect you to be an expert on. Complete these tasks, which build an answer to each research question, carefully and neatly because they will become your revision notes. Many tasks use tables – give yourself room – each table should have its own page.

> **?** If you have gaps in your knowledge, go back to your research notes and the relevant section of this book and make sure that you add anything that is missing so you have covered all the key topics in enough detail.

Summarise

Turns your learning into a **memorable form**. Sometimes we guide you to do this, but mostly it is up to you.

Memory aids are different from your research notes. They use images or diagrams, but very few words. Most people remember better if something is summarised with both text and visuals.

> **?** If you cannot remember some of the content you have covered, go back to your research notes and improve or recreate your memory aid.

Reflect

These tasks make you form **connections** between what you have already learned and what you are about to learn.

Apply ▶ Recall Challenge

Prepare yourself for exams by testing yourself on what you have learned.

Quizzes, games and competitions test how much you can remember. They identify your weak spots where you need to spend more time.

> **?** If you did not understand how to approach a question, go back to the Exam Tips in this book and re-read them, checking you fully understand what is required in a good answer to that type of question.

Apply ▶ Exam Practice

Continue to prepare for the exam by answering exam-style questions with our Exam Tips to guide you.

Our **practice questions** are like the questions you will be asked in the exam, although none of them come from actual past papers. You can get real papers from your teacher or from the AQA website. There are **Exam Tips** for each question type – showing you how to approach it.

Review

We regularly **review** the **big ideas and concepts**. We also encourage you to **review your own learning** regularly.

> **Take responsibility** **?** Review your own learning. What areas did you do well on? What areas do you need to improve?

Revision Tips

1. **Don't delay** revision until just before the exam
   Revision should be an ongoing process. You need to revisit topics that you have studied regularly. Otherwise, as the graph shows, you will quickly start to forget key topics.
2. **Retrieval practice** makes your memory stronger
   When you recall what you have previously studied, your brain strengthens connections and makes it easier to recall this information in the future.
3. **Spaced practice** helps you remember for longer!
   At the end of each topic, we test you, not just on that topic but on previous ones as well. You should regularly return to the Review tasks from previous topics and test your knowledge of 'older material'. As the graph shows, this should improve recall and stop you forgetting.

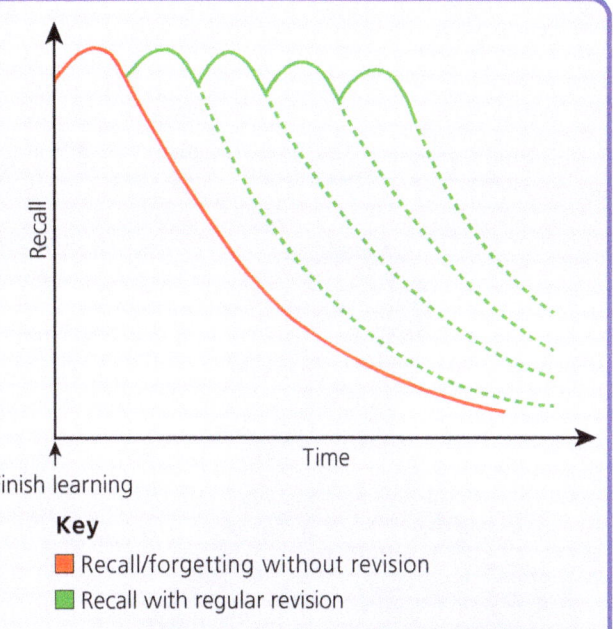

Key
- Recall/forgetting without revision
- Recall with regular revision

Apply ▶ Recall Challenge

1 Know your individuals

Match each person below with the correct description.

Individual	How their work influenced the development of medicine
Galen	Developed a vaccination against smallpox
Vesalius	Developed the Germ Theory
Harvey	Wrote a report recommending the setting up of the National Health Service
Paré	Described how the heart acts as a pump and circulates blood around the body
Jenner	A Roman doctor whose books influenced medicine in the medieval and Renaissance periods
Pasteur	Produced a book called *The Fabrica* which accurately described the structure of the body (anatomy)
Beveridge	Improved surgical techniques during the Renaissance period

2 Know your key words

Match each key word below with its definition or description.

Key words	Definition
Antibiotics	An event that killed nearly half the population of England during the Middle Ages
Antiseptics	A belief that people became ill because liquids in the body were out of balance
Anaesthetics	The injection into the body of killed or weakened organisms to give the body resistance against the disease
The NHS	Chemicals used to destroy bacteria and prevent infection
The four humours	A group of drugs used to treat and cure infections caused by bacteria
The Black Death	A drug given to produce unconsciousness before and during surgery
Vaccinations	Set up in 1948 to provide free health care to everyone

Period introduction: The Middle Ages

1.1 Introducing ... Claudius Galen

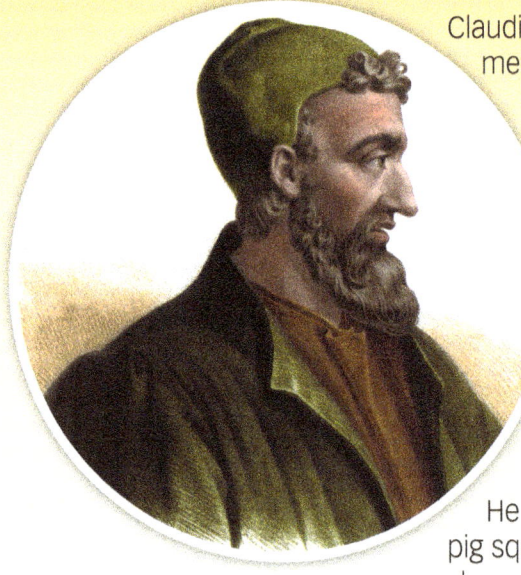

Claudius Galen was born in Greece in AD129 and began studying medicine when he was just 16 years old.

At the age of 20, he moved to Rome where he soon made a reputation for himself as a doctor. He became doctor for the Roman Emperor and his family.

The squealing pig

Galen was a great showman. He would do public **dissections** of animals and give talks.

In one famous performance, Galen showed his discoveries about the nervous system by dissecting a pig. As the pig squealed on the table, he cut into its neck, finding the nerves.

He could have cut through the correct nerve to stop the pig squealing immediately, but that did not appeal to Galen's showmanship. Instead, he announced, 'I will cut this nerve but the pig will keep squealing.' He cut, and the pig kept squealing. He cut again, building up the tension, and again the pig kept squealing.

Finally he announced, 'When I cut this nerve, the pig will stop squealing.' He cut and the pig was silent!

Books, books and more books

Galen wrote more than 350 books which covered every aspect of medicine. These were extremely detailed and well organised. They combined old Greek ideas (for example, the Theory of the Four Humours) with what he had learned from his own work.

It seemed as if Galen had covered everything so thoroughly that people believed his books contained all the answers. They became the basis for medical training for the next 1500 years.

People in the Middle Ages respected traditional ideas, so few tried to suggest alternative theories about what caused disease or how to treat it.

The support of the Church

One key reason Galen's books lasted so long was that his ideas fitted in with the ideas of the Christian Church, which controlled education in Europe in the Middle Ages.

Galen was not a Christian, but he taught that the body had been created by one god, who had made all the parts of the body fit together perfectly. This matched the Christian belief that God had created human beings.

> **Reflect**
>
> **Why did a doctor from Roman times still influence doctors 1500 years later?**
>
> 1 Record at least three reasons why Galen's work still influenced doctors in the Middle Ages.
> 2 Identify which of the following areas of medicine Galen influenced:
>   a Knowledge of the cause of disease
>   b Treatments
>   c Ways of preventing illness
>   d Public health
>   e Surgery

What were the key features of 'Galenic medicine'?

Before Galen

- A Greek doctor called Hippocrates was the main influence on medical ideas.
- Hippocrates taught that people got ill because their humours were out of balance (see information panel).
- He taught doctors to examine patients carefully and to keep detailed notes of symptoms.

Galen's old ideas – building on Hippocrates

- Galen also believed that people became sick when their humours were out of balance.
- He also recommended exercise and a good diet to stay healthy.
- His most common treatments were bleeding or making people vomit to restore the balance of the humours.

Galen's new ideas

The Theory of Opposites: Galen developed the idea of using 'opposites' to balance the humours. For example, if a patient had too much phlegm, then the illness was caused by cold. Galen's treatment was the opposite – he gave the patient a hot food such as peppers.

Galen's discoveries in anatomy were important. He proved that:
- the brain, not the heart, controlled speech
- the arteries, and not just the veins, carried blood around the body.

Dissection and knowledge of the body: Galen believed that physicians (doctors) should find out as much as possible about the body (anatomy). If possible, they should dissect human bodies themselves. If this was not possible, Galen told them to dissect apes because they were most like humans.

But... LIMITATIONS

He made mistakes because the bodies of apes and pigs are not the same as humans. Some of his mistakes went unchallenged for over a thousand years.

Long-term significance (the next 1500 years!)

Because he wrote such good books, and had the support of the Church, doctors followed Galen's ideas for the next 1500 years.

The Theory of the Four Humours

This theory taught that:
- The body contains four humours or liquids (blood, phlegm, yellow bile and black bile).
- People became sick because they had too much or too little of one humour.
- For good health, humours needed to be balanced, so doctors gave advice on what to eat (diet) and how to exercise to stay in balance. They also bled patients or made them vomit to restore balance.
- People followed this theory because it made sense of the symptoms they observed. For example, a sick person might vomit yellow bile, or sneeze phlegm or bleed from the nose. This suggested that the body was unbalanced and was trying to get rid of too much of one humour.
- They also followed it because the advice on diet and exercise did work. Nowadays, we know that a balanced diet and lots of exercise make you healthier. It was the same then.

Revision Tip

A good memory aid summarises the key points in as few words as possible. This example shows how key words and images can help trigger memory so that you can recall the key features of Galenic medicine.

The 5Bs of Galenic medicine

 **B**alance the 4 humours

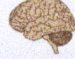 **B**rain controls speech

 Blood carried by arteries and veins

 Body structure of humans like apes

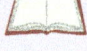 **B**ooks influence medicine for over 1500 years

Topic 1: Medieval medicine

1.2 Beliefs about the causes of illness and methods of prevention and treatment in the Middle Ages

Research & Record

How did ideas about the causes of disease influence methods of prevention and treatment?

Use pages 14 and 15 to complete your own copy of a table like this. Record examples of prevention and treatment linked to each of the main ideas.

Ideas about cause	Methods of prevention and treatment
A punishment from God	People said prayers while they made herbal remedies
Bad air	
Astrology	
Superstition	
Unbalanced humours	

Beliefs about the causes of illness and disease

A punishment from God

The most common belief was that God sent illnesses to punish people for their sins. For example, one churchman said the plague was a punishment for children who did not respect their parents.

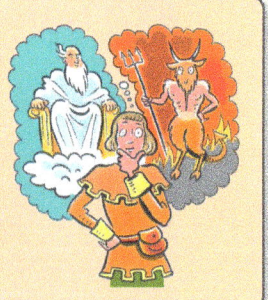

Bad air

A common explanation was that bad air caused illness. Some people linked the bad air to filth in the streets but could not explain what the link was.

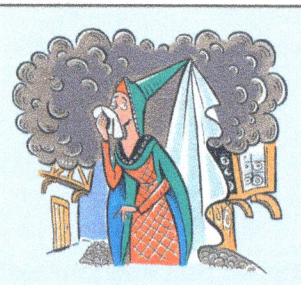

Astrology

Illness was sometimes linked to the movement of the planets and *astrology*.

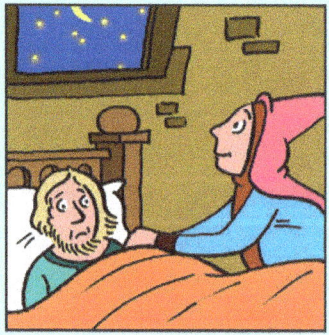

Unbalanced humours

Hippocrates and Galen taught that people got ill when their humours were out of balance. British and European physicians had been trained using Galen's books, so they believed the same. Islamic doctors also believed in the importance of the four humours because they studied Galen's books. This explanation was based on Hippocrates' observations of what happened when people were sick – they got rid of the excess humour.

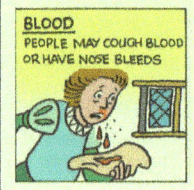
BLOOD PEOPLE MAY COUGH BLOOD OR HAVE NOSE BLEEDS

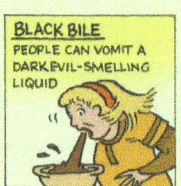
BLACK BILE PEOPLE CAN VOMIT A DARK EVIL-SMELLING LIQUID

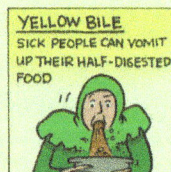
YELLOW BILE SICK PEOPLE CAN VOMIT UP THEIR HALF-DIGESTED FOOD

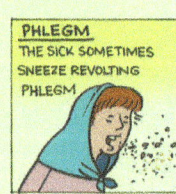
PHLEGM THE SICK SOMETIMES SNEEZE REVOLTING PHLEGM

Preventing, diagnosing and treating illness

Urine chart
The physician used a chart like this to test a patient's urine. The chart shows the colour, smell and thickness of urine. The doctor might also have tasted the urine. Inspecting urine was a vital part of diagnosing an illness. This method of diagnosis was called 'uroscopy' and was one way to judge if a patient's humours were in balance. For example, very white urine was seen as a sign of too much phlegm in the body.

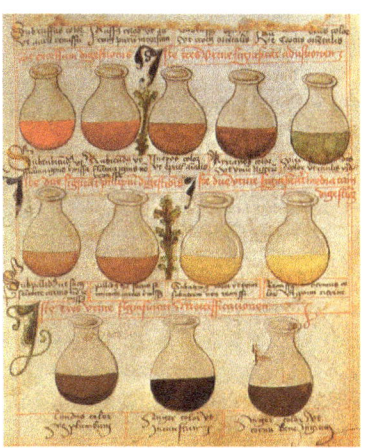

Zodiac man

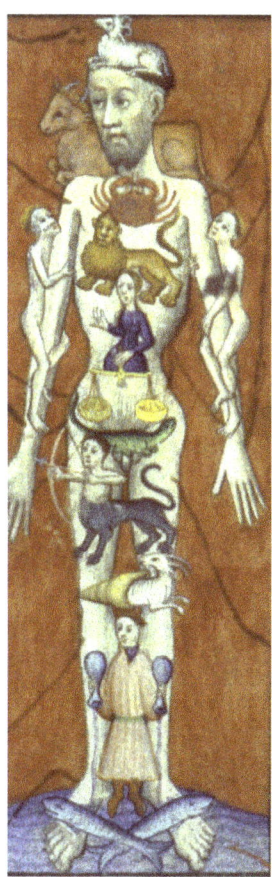

Doctors believed that the movement of the Sun, moon and planets through the constellations (groups of stars) affected people's bodies. The zodiac chart showed the doctor when (and when not) to treat each part of the body. For example, when the moon was passing through Pisces (the fish), the doctor should not treat the patient's feet.

Bleeding
People were bled regularly to avoid illness. Bleeding was done by a surgeon or doctor. The picture below shows a doctor balancing his patient's humours by letting blood flow from his arm. Alternatively, leeches were used to bite into the patient and suck out the blood.
In some monasteries, monks were bled seven to twelve times per year to prevent illness. Sometimes the monk was bled to the point of unconsciousness – which means he probably lost three or four pints of blood!

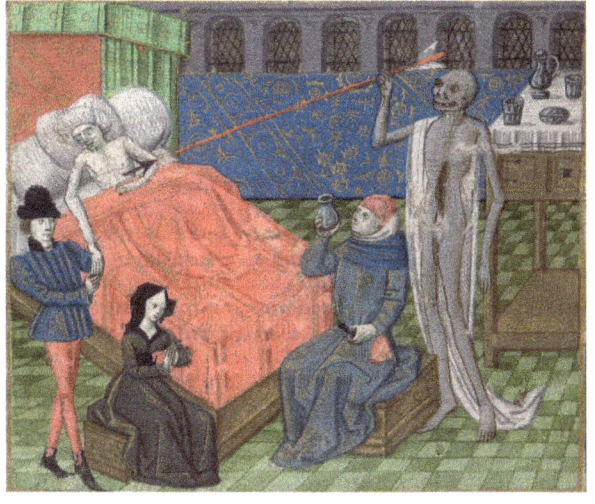

Cleaning the streets
In 1349, plague struck London. King Edward III ordered the Lord Mayor to remove all the filth lying in the streets. He wrote that 'the filth from the houses is infecting the air, endangering people through the sickness which is increasing daily.'

Herbal remedies
The most common remedies were made from herbs, minerals and animal parts. Most women knew them by heart, but they also were written down in books called 'herbals', with pictures of the ingredients and explanations of the exact quantities of each ingredient and how to mix the potion. They also included prayers to say while collecting the herbs to increase the effectiveness of the remedy.

1.3 The medieval doctor

> ### Research & Record
> **Who treated sick people and how were they trained?**
> Use the information on pages 16–17 to make notes about:
> 1. who treated sick people in the Middle Ages
> 2. how the healers were trained.

Physicians

Physicians were the highest-ranking doctors. They were well-paid. Only the rich could afford to go to a physician. They treated kings, nobles and wealthy merchants.

There were very few physicians. In the 1300s, there were less than 100 physicians in England.

Treatments

Physicians used a range of treatments based on the Theory of the Four Humours. As well as bleeding or purging, they would advise patients how to stay healthy by regular washing, cleaning teeth, combing hair, exercising in the fresh air and bathing in hot water.

Training

Physicians were trained at university. Source 1 shows one part of student physicians' training – watching a dissection.

The physician (on the right) was in charge but did not do the dissection. He told the surgeon which part of the body to dissect. He also told his assistant (middle right) which passages of Galen to read out to illustrate the dissection. The students had to listen to Galen's words and watch the dissection. They were not allowed to do anything!

The dissections were designed to show that Galen's descriptions of the body were correct. They were not investigations to make new discoveries. Physicians believed that Galen's books contained everything they needed to learn about the human body.

▼ **SOURCE 1** Training for medieval doctors

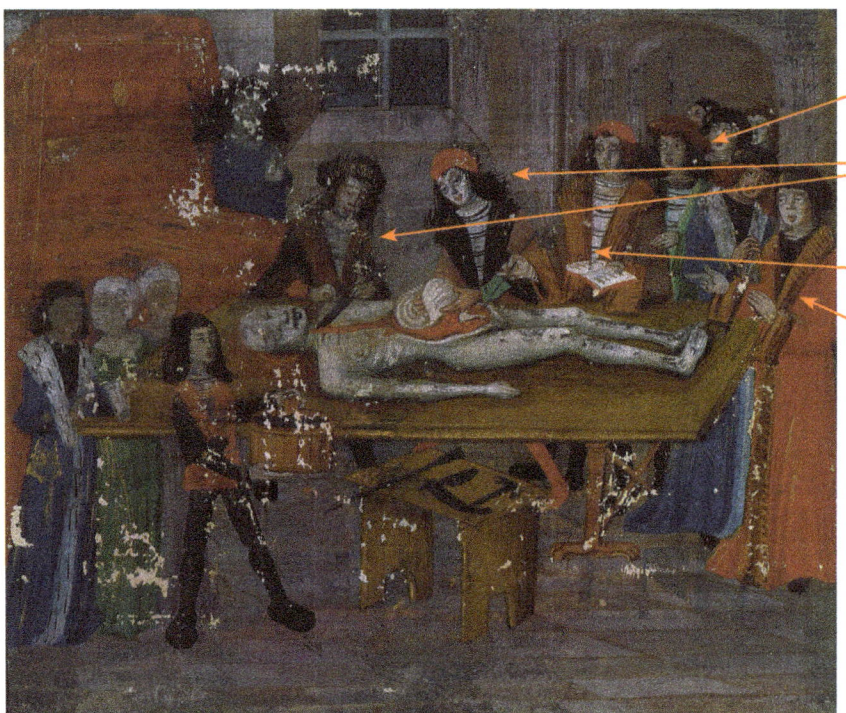

- Students – watching and listening
- Surgeons – doing the dissection
- Assistant – reading Galen out loud
- Physician – in charge

Women

Most people could not afford a physician, so they were treated at home by a member of their family – usually a woman.

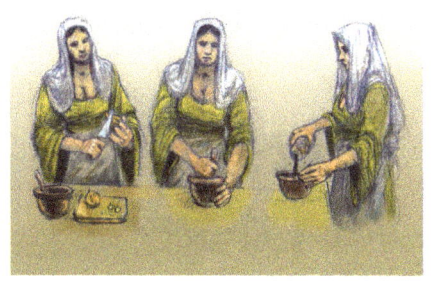

Most women would have learned a wide range of remedies from their mother or grandmother and they used these to treat their husbands and children. There might also be a wise woman in the village who they could consult when they did not know how to treat an illness.

Remedies were not just **superstition**. They sometimes worked. For example, many included honey which is known to fight infection.

Women also acted as midwives. In some towns, midwives had to serve an apprenticeship to learn the 'trade' and gain a licence to practice, and were then paid for their expertise.

Surgeons

If you had a little money and were very worried about your illness, you might see a local surgeon. Some surgeons were skilful because they had been trained as apprentices to experienced surgeons. There was a guild of master surgeons which required new members to gain licences by passing tests. Some surgeons read books by great European surgeons, such as **Guy de Chauliac**. Women could qualify as surgeons by working as apprentices. You will find out more about surgeons on page 22.

Summarise

Create memory aids to remember key features

A good memory aid:
- answers a key question
- uses minimal words – just key words
- includes a memorable image, diagram or mnemonic.

Here is an example to summarise the information on pages 14–17.

1. Copy the memory aid and add notes to the 4BAG mnemonic so it is ready to be used for revision.
2. Complete the bullet points to summarise the role of women in medicine.

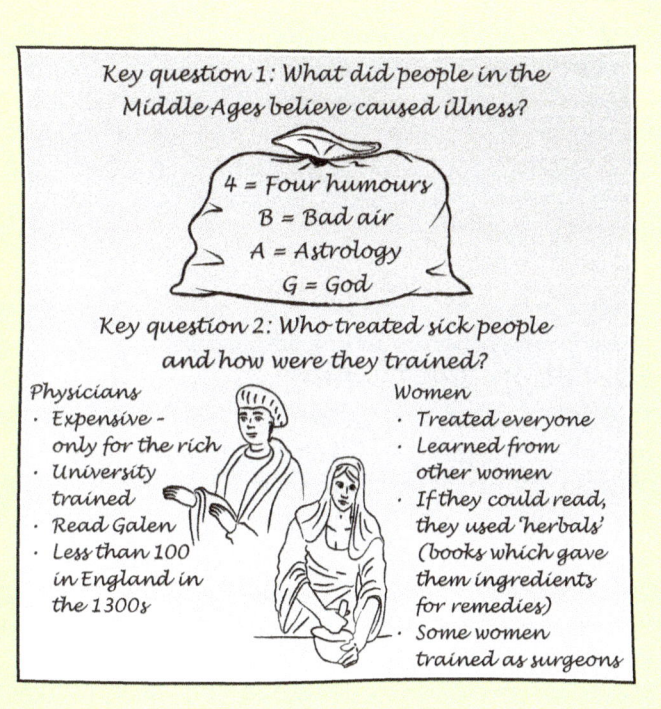

Topic 2: Medical progress in the Middle Ages

2.1 The contribution of Christianity to medical progress and treatment

Research & Record

How far did Christian religion help medicine progress?

Read pages 18 and 19 and complete a table like this, showing how Christianity influenced medicine in both a positive and a negative way.

Area of medicine	Positive: How did religion help medicine?	Negative: How did religion hinder medicine?
Preserving knowledge	Made sure people could learn from Greek and Roman ideas	
Education and training		Taught to follow Galen and not to question ideas
Ideas about the causes of disease and treatments		
Caring for sick people		

Preserving knowledge

The collapse of the Roman Empire nearly destroyed the medical knowledge that had been built up by the Greeks and the Romans. However, two religions, Christianity and Islam, made sure this knowledge was not lost. They saved many Greek and Roman medical books from destruction. Monks in Christian monasteries made copies of ancient books, by hand, including books by Galen and other medical writers.

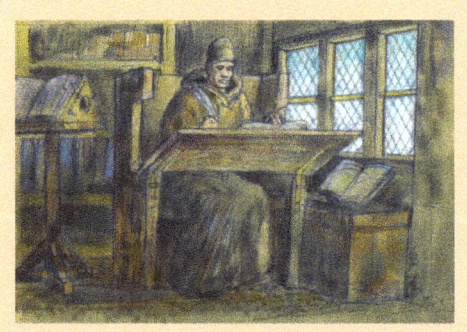

Education and training

The Christian Church controlled the universities where physicians trained. They made sure that physicians read and trusted the work of Galen. The Church liked Galen because his teaching supported the Christian idea that God had created human beings.

Physicians were not encouraged by the Church to challenge traditional ideas. If people started questioning Galen's teachings, they might question the Bible too, so questioning was not a good idea! When Roger Bacon said that doctors should do their own research instead of just reading Galen, he was put in prison by Church leaders.

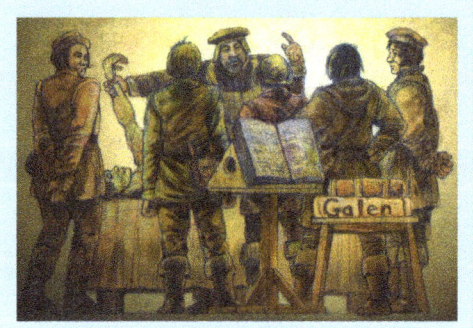

Ideas about the causes of disease and treatments

Christian teaching also influenced people's ideas about what caused disease. The Bible said that God controlled all aspects of life, so it was logical that God also sent disease. But why would God send disease? Many believed it was as punishment for their sins. This had two results:

- If God sent diseases, this meant that there was no need to look for other causes. This was an important reason why ideas about what caused disease did not change.
- If disease was a punishment for sin, then there was also no need to look for other treatments. You just had to be more religious, pray more and commit fewer sins.

This control of ideas extended all the way from the Pope in Rome, through the archbishops and bishops, to the priest in every village in medieval Britain. This network allowed the Church to influence everyone's ideas.

Hospitals

The Christian Church also taught that sick people should be looked after. This led to many hospitals being founded in the Middle Ages.

Patients: Medieval hospitals functioned more like care homes do today – they mostly looked after those living in poverty and older people. However, a person could not get into a hospital if they had a disease that other people might catch!

Nurses: Nursing care was usually provided by nuns.

Treatments: The patients were given food and rest. The nuns also provided herbal remedies, often taken from the books in their library. However, the most important treatment was prayer. At the end of each ward there was an altar where priests said mass seven times each day. The patients joined in the prayers, hoping that God would forgive their sins. Christian saints were also linked to particular illnesses, so people would pray for help from that saint.

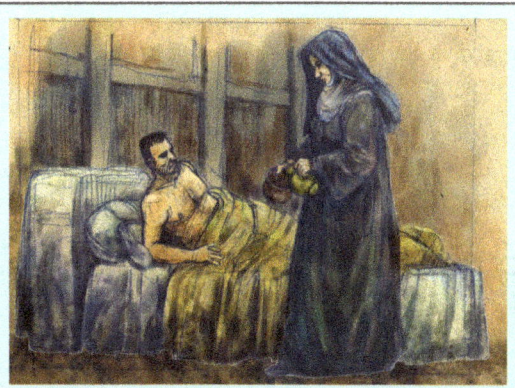

By 1400, there were nearly 500 hospitals in England. Most were very small, with an average of about ten patients. There were also some specialist hospitals.

In London, Richard Whittington, the Lord Mayor, paid for an eight-bed hospital for unmarried pregnant women.

In Chester, there was a hospital for the care of 'poor and silly persons'.

Leper houses were built outside towns to separate those with **leprosy** from healthy people.

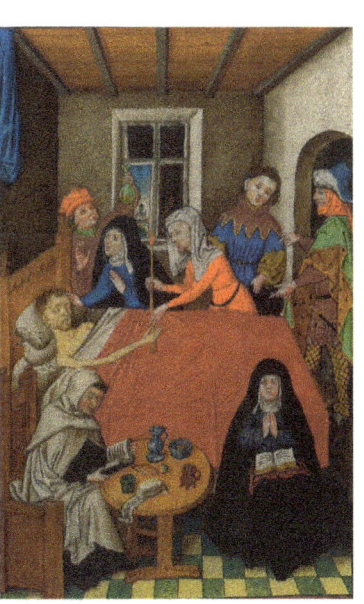

▶ **SOURCE 1** A deathbed scene from a prayer book called *The Hours of Catherine of Cleves* painted in around 1400. The doctor is examining the patient's urine. At the same time, people are praying for the patient. The lighted candle is to help the dying man's soul get to heaven

Reflect

1. Why is Source 1 useful for a historian studying medicine in the Middle Ages?
2. What religious treatments does it show?
3. What other approaches to diagnosing and treating illness does it show?

2.2 The nature and importance of Islamic medicine

Research & Record

How did Islamic scholars and doctors influence the development of medicine in Europe?

Complete an argument bridge like this to show how Islamic scholars and doctors played an important role in the development of medicine in Britain and the rest of Europe.

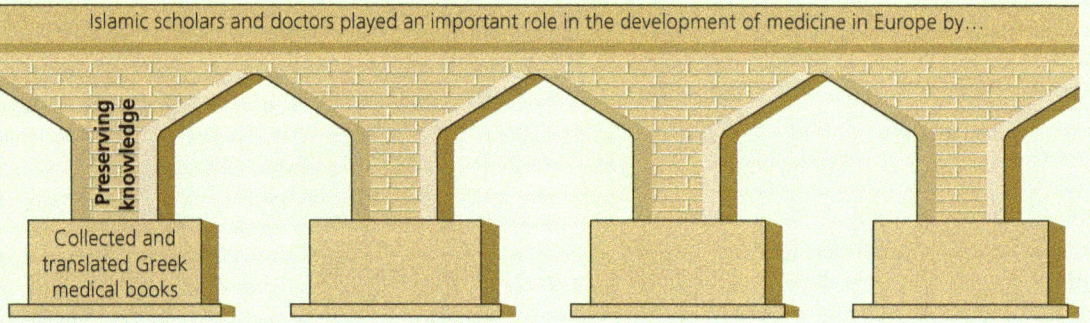

Hospitals

Islamic teachings encouraged people to take care of their diet, exercise and hygiene. Islam also encouraged people to care for those who were sick or in need. One result of this was the development of hospitals.

The first Islamic hospital was founded in Baghdad around AD805 and by the 1100s, every large town in the Islamic world had a hospital.

Hospitals and medical schools were funded by wealthy individuals. The hospitals were open to all, organised into wards and provided nursing care for patients. Physicians were trained at these hospitals.

The hospital at Cairo, built in 1283, had specialist wards for mental and physical disorders, plus a surgery, pharmacy, library and lecture rooms for teaching. There was both a mosque and a Christian chapel.

Preserving knowledge

Islamic physicians built on the ideas of the Ancient Greeks and Romans.

Many Greek medical books were translated into Arabic by Islamic scholars. The city of Baghdad was the main centre for collecting and translating medical texts. Without these translations, the books by Galen and others could well have been lost.

Islamic doctors wrote multi-volume medical encyclopedias which organised medical knowledge with great thoroughness. They included the work of Galen and other Greek medical writers. These books were later translated from Arabic into Latin and were used in Europe so that European physicians learned more about the work of Galen and Arab doctors.

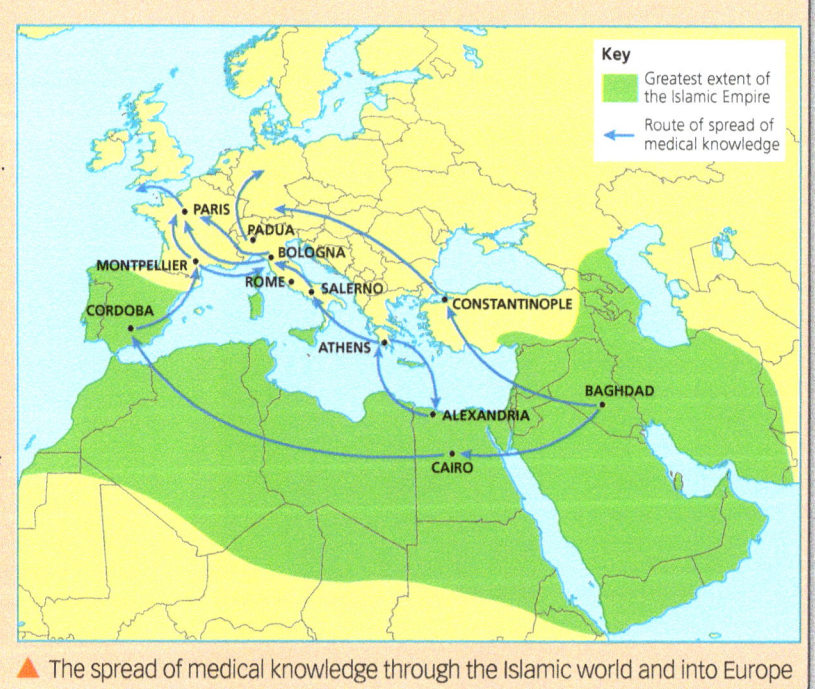

▲ The spread of medical knowledge through the Islamic world and into Europe

> **Revision Tip**
>
> **Use argument bridges to help you write better answers in the exam**
>
> Argument bridges help you organise your ideas and make sure that your arguments are fully supported by clear points and strong evidence. This is crucial for success in the exam.
> - Your overall argument is like a bridge that needs supporting pillars and strong foundations. If the pillars are not strong or there are no foundations, the bridge crumbles.
> - The supporting pillars are the key ideas that you will consider as part of your argument.
> - The foundations are the supporting evidence. They are the specific examples which create a strong foundation for each pillar.

Key individuals

Islamic doctors had a great influence on medicine in Western Europe. As well as preserving the ideas of the Ancient Greeks and Romans, Islamic physicians added their own research. For example, they developed new techniques for treating cataracts and other eye complaints.

The work of these key individuals was translated into Latin and used in medical schools to train physicians.

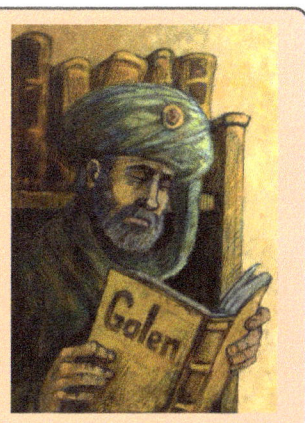

Al-Razi (or Rhazes)
- Wrote over 50 books based on the ideas of Hippocrates and Galen, as well as Chinese and Indian sources.
- His books were used for centuries after his death in AD925.
- His books emphasised the importance of the physician carefully diagnosing the illness.
- He also described smallpox and measles accurately.

Ibn-al-Nafis
- Argued against Galen's theory that blood was produced in the liver and burnt up in the body as a nutrient.
- Instead, he argued that blood circulated around the body.

Al-Zahrawi (or Albucasis)
- Was a well-known expert in surgery.
- Produced a book describing complex abdominal operations and showing illustrations of more than 200 surgical instruments.

Ibn Sina (or Avicenna)
- Encouraged observation and experimentation, as well as emphasising the importance of clean air and water.
- Wrote on a wide range of topics. His most important books were *The Book of Healing* and *The Cannon of Medicine*.
- *The Cannon of Medicine* became the main medical textbook for physicians until the seventeenth century. It described, for example, over 700 drugs and medicines and their uses, and how to diagnose diseases.

2.3 Surgery in medieval times

Research & Record

In what areas did surgery progress, 1000–1500?
There was clear progress in surgery during the medieval period. However, medieval surgeons still struggled to overcome many problems.

Use the case studies and information boxes on these two pages to gather examples under both headings.

Ways that surgery progressed
- Surgeons developed forceps to remove arrowheads

Way that surgery did not progress
- Surgeons struggled to stop infections spreading

Treatments

Most surgery was performed by 'barber-surgeons'. They offered blood-letting, tooth extractions and **amputations**, as well as haircuts and shaves! They could also remove small tumours on the skin's surface.

Surgeons could not do complex operations inside the body. They did not know enough anatomy and they faced the surgeon's three problems: pain, infection and bleeding.

The surgeon's three problems

Pain: Occasionally surgeons had to amputate a limb or remove painful bladder stones without any pain relief. Imagine the pain the patient felt! Surgeons used herbs such as opium or hemlock to make patients drowsy, but risked putting the patient to sleep permanently!

Infection: Wine, vinegar or honey were used to clean wounds, but they could not prevent infections spreading.

Bleeding: Large cuts were sewn up and often **cauterised** (see Source 1). Surgeons could not stop heavy bleeding.

Training

Surgeons did not go to university but trained as apprentices through observing others. They improved their skills through practice and reading books on surgery (see Source 1).

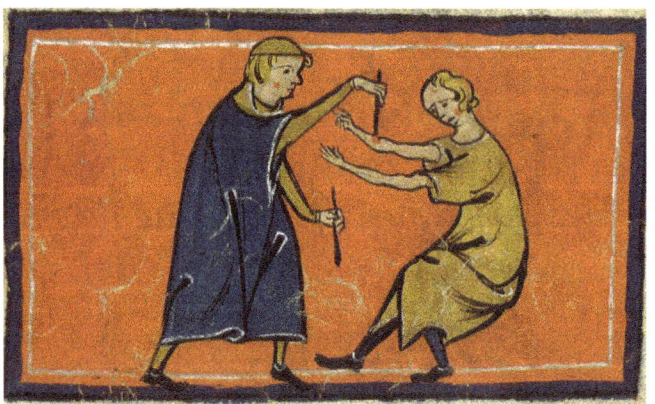

▶ **SOURCE 1** An illustration from a surgical book. This shows cauterising, a common method of closing wounds by sealing them with a burning iron. It would not be much help to a surgeon to know how to do it!

Case study A: Saving the Prince's life

16-year-old Henry, Prince of Wales, lay wounded on the battlefield. An arrow had passed through his cheek and lodged in the bottom of his skull. The royal surgeon, John Bradmore, knew he had to remove the arrowhead. Any pieces left in the wound would poison and kill the Prince.

Bradmore designed a new forcep which could pass through the cheek wound to take hold of the arrowhead and remove it.

For the next three weeks, he carefully dressed the wound with barley and honey. It healed, free from any infection.

This is one example of how war led to improvements in surgery. Surgeons had to develop new techniques to solve the problems they faced on the battlefields.

Case study B: Disagreeing with Galen

Everyday experience led some to disagree with Galen. He taught that wounds were more likely to heal if pus developed, believing the pus carried away poisoned blood that caused infection. Doctors therefore covered wounds in ointments and bandages designed to make pus develop.

Henri de Mondeville (c1260–c1320) was an army surgeon and teacher who disagreed with this method. He taught his students to bathe and cleanse wounds, then close them up quickly, without trying to form pus. We now know this is much more likely to lead to successful healing.

Exam Tip

Use connectives and evidence for stronger arguments

When arguing the importance of a factor, you have to prove it was important. For example:

Communication was an important factor that helped medicine progress during the medieval period. Books were produced by Islamic doctors that preserved knowledge from the Ancient Greeks and included new ideas about the way the body worked. This meant that doctors in Britain and other parts of Europe could learn ideas from other cultures. For example, Avicenna's medical encyclopedia, *The Canon*, was used to teach European physicians until the 1600s. In addition, surgeons in Britain had access to carefully illustrated books on surgical techniques. This led to the spread of surgical techniques and old ideas, such as the belief that pus helped wounds heal, being challenged. Guy de Chauliac wrote a seven-volume book on surgery and this demonstrates the detailed knowledge that medieval surgeons could draw on to develop their surgical skills.

Use connectives to tie what you know to the question

Phrases like 'this meant that', 'this led to', and 'this resulted in' are called connectives because they tie what you know to the question and so help you prove your argument.

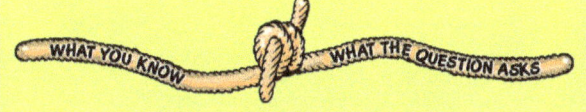

Add specific examples

Provide evidence to substantiate (support) your argument. Use phrases such as 'for example', 'such as' and 'this demonstrates' to introduce or flag your supporting evidence.

Apply ▶ Exam Practice

Use the Exam Tip to complete two developed arguments.

1. The first paragraph should prove the importance of warfare in improvements in surgery. You can base that on what you have read on these two pages.

2. The second should prove the importance of religion in the development of hospitals. You can base that on what you learned on pages 18–21.

Topic 3: Public health in the Middle Ages

3.1 Towns and monasteries

> ### Research & Record
> **What public health problems existed in medieval towns?**
> 1. As the information below shows, medieval people did want their towns to be clean. However, despite some improvements, public health problems remained. How many can you find in Source 1?
> 2. Use Source 2, on the opposite page, to record three features that show how and why health facilities were better in monasteries.

Public health problems

- Water for drinking or cooking was collected from a river or storage pit.
- **Cesspits** for human waste were sometimes built near water supplies.
- People threw rubbish (including human excrement) into the streets and rivers.
- Cattle, sheep and geese roamed the streets. Horses were used as transport. These animals left dung.
- Diseases such as plague were common and spread very quickly.
- Open sewers or drains ran through the streets.

Public health improvements

- Night carts collected human waste from cesspits.
- Rakers were sent to clean the streets.
- In Exeter, aqueducts were built to bring fresh water to the town.
- In Newcastle, streets were paved to make them drier and easier to clean.
- Cesspits were lined with brick or stone so they did not leak into water supplies.
- Laws were passed to punish people for throwing human or butchers' waste into the street.

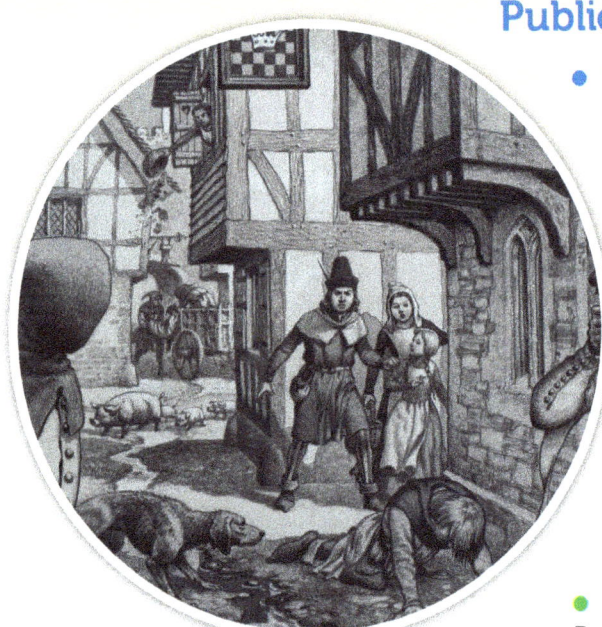

▲ **SOURCE 1** An artist's impression of a London street in the Middle Ages. From *Look and Learn* magazine, 1976

Public health in monasteries

The best public health facilities were in monasteries for three main reasons.

- Monasteries were wealthy. Rich people gave them money in return for prayers. Their wealth allowed monasteries to install water supplies and sanitation.
- Monasteries were often close to rivers, built in isolated places where they drew fresh water.
- Monks were expected to keep clean. They washed their clothes regularly. Some monks had a bath once a month.

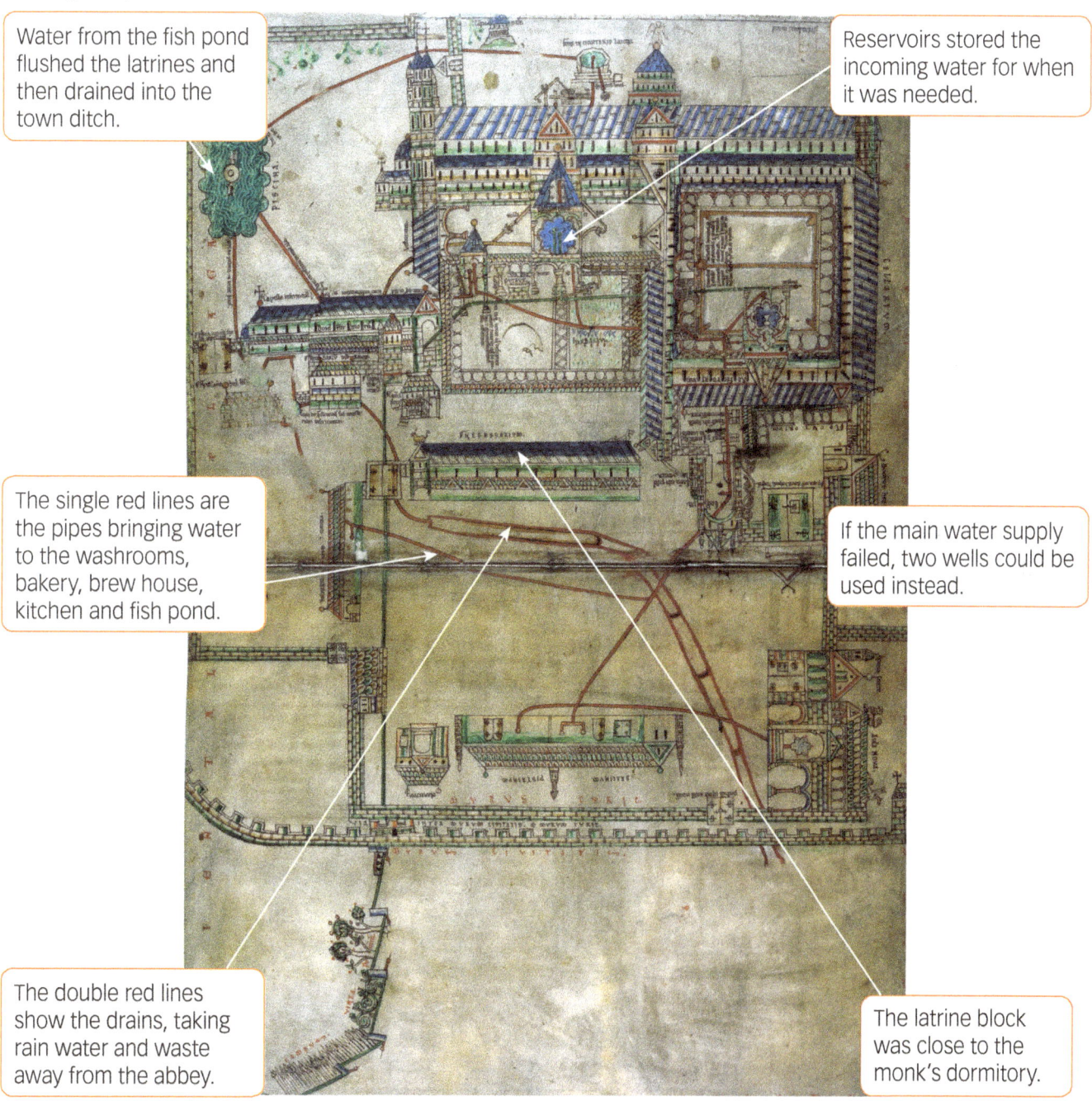

Water from the fish pond flushed the latrines and then drained into the town ditch.

Reservoirs stored the incoming water for when it was needed.

The single red lines are the pipes bringing water to the washrooms, bakery, brew house, kitchen and fish pond.

If the main water supply failed, two wells could be used instead.

The double red lines show the drains, taking rain water and waste away from the abbey.

The latrine block was close to the monk's dormitory.

▲ **SOURCE 2** A plan of the water system at Canterbury Abbey, drawn by the engineer who designed it in the 1100s

3.2 Case study: The Black Death in Britain

Research & Record

What can the Black Death tell us about medicine and public health in medieval Britain?

We can learn a lot about medicine in the medieval period from a case study of the Black Death. Use the information on pages 26–27 to complete your own copy of this table.

Black Death facts		
When did the Black Death arrive in England?	What percentage of people in Britain died?	What were buboes?
Which **two** diseases do historians think were involved?	Which **two** animals/insects probably spread the disease?	List **two** long-term consequences of the disease.
List **three** methods of prevention linked to the idea that God had caused the Black Death.	List **three** methods of prevention linked to the idea that bad air caused the Black Death.	Give **three** examples of how people tried to treat the disease.

Causes: What was the Black Death?

The Black Death was one of the most frightening diseases in history. The map shows how it spread across Europe after arriving from Asia.

It reached England in 1348. Over the next twelve months, historians estimate that the Black Death killed over one-third of the population. Towns and ports were hardest hit. Only remote villages and farms avoided it. The plague affected both rich and poor.

Judging by the way the symptoms were described, historians think the Black Death was a combination of two diseases. The **main disease** was bubonic plague, carried by rats and spread by fleas. People with the disease felt cold and tired, then got painful swellings called **buboes**, as big as eggs, on their neck and in their groin or armpits. These were quickly followed by high fever, severe headache, then usually death after three days.

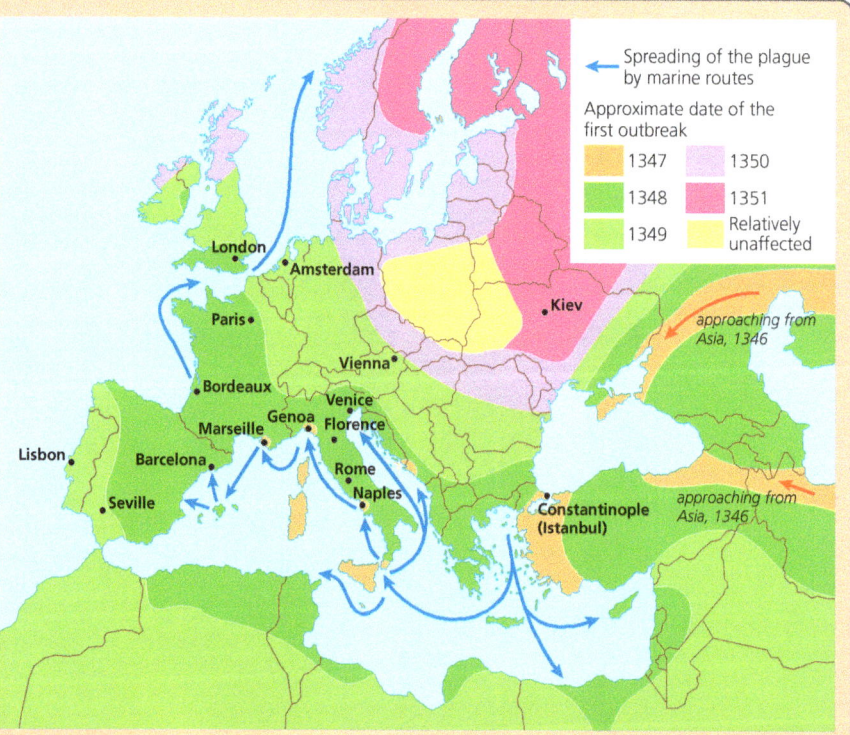

The **epidemic** was probably made worse by pneumonic plague. This was spread by people coughing over others. The disease attacked the lungs. People then coughed up blood. They died more quickly from this plague than from bubonic plague – in a day or two at most.

Explanations: What did people at the time believe caused it?

God's punishment – the plague was part of God's plan to make people less sinful.
Miasma – bad, stinking air (called 'miasma') coming from rubbish in the streets spread disease.
Astrology – people became ill because a planet had moved into a new constellation of stars.
The Theory of the Four Humours – people died because they were 'stuffed with evil humours'.

Prevention: How did people try to prevent it from spreading?

There were many different methods. Here is a selection.

- People stopped strangers entering their villages in case they carried the plague.
- Bishops ordered daily services and processions to pray for forgiveness and ask for God's help.
- King Edward III wrote to the Mayor of London, ordering him to clean the streets. He said that the rubbish was creating 'bad odours' that led to the disease spreading.
- Butchers were punished for leaving the remains of slaughtered animals in the streets.
- People lit huge candles in church as offerings to God.
- People fasted (stopped eating) to show they were sorry for their sins.
- Doors and windows were shut and sealed.
- People went on pilgrimages to pray for God's forgiveness at the tombs of saints.
- People carried sweet-smelling herbs or lit fires to overpower the bad air.
- People kept the air moving by ringing bells or keeping birds to fly around the house.
- Activities that might be insulting to God were ended. For example, in Suffolk they stopped using churchyards for wrestling matches.
- Some people punished themselves in public and begged God for forgiveness, as you can see in Source 1 below.

▼ **SOURCE 1** This picture shows the Flagellants who arrived in London from Holland. According to the chronicler Robert of Avebury, they walked barefoot through the city twice a day, wearing only a linen cloth. They whipped themselves to show God they had repented their sins and asked God to be merciful

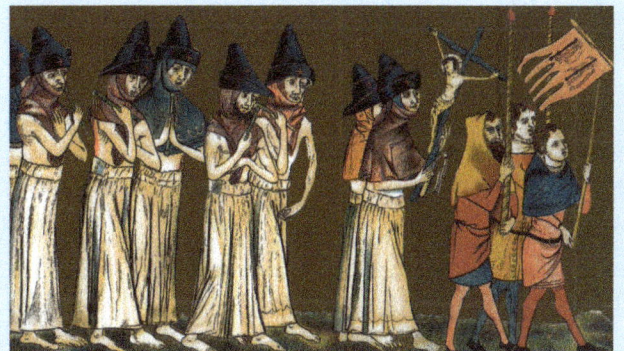

Treatments: How did people treat the disease?

- They prayed for people to recover.
- They put holy charms round the necks of sick people.
- They cut open the buboes to let out the pus.
- They used leeches to bleed the patients.
- They tried treatments based on Galen's 'treatment by opposites'. As the Black Death was a fever, cold foods and baths were used and people were told to avoid hot (strong) foods such as garlic and onions.

Impact: What were the consequences?

In the short term: The Black Death killed over one-third of the population of medieval England in a year. Whole villages were wiped out. The loss of so many workers led to food shortages. Food prices increased.

In the long term: Survivors became better-off. There was a shortage of workers, so employers had to pay higher wages to attract them. People had more money and spent some of this on education. More people learned to read and write, which helped to spread new ideas more quickly.

3.3 Middle Ages period review

> ### Review 1
> #### Themes
> 1. The period summary chart below summarises the medieval period. Study it carefully, then create a blank copy (with only the themes listed on the left-hand side) and try to reproduce all the information **from memory alone**. Use a whole page of A4 paper with 6 rows – one per theme. This is a challenge but worth the effort because it will reveal what you are able to remember easily and what you are finding harder to recall.
> 2. Once you have done the best you can, review your attempt against our period summary chart. Fill in any gaps using a **different colour pen**. This will remind you what you are struggling to remember.

Period summary, c1000–1500	
Theme	**Health and the people in the Middle Ages, c1000–1500**
Ideas about the cause of illness	• Four humours – blood, black bile, yellow bile and phlegm unbalanced • Bad air (miasma) • Astrology – movement of the planets • God – a punishment for sins
Knowledge of the human body	• Doctors followed the ideas of Galen • Knew about Greek, Roman and Arab discoveries • Doctors encouraged to accept traditional ideas – not make new discoveries • Dissections were done to illustrate what Galen had said
Treatments	• Prayers and charms • Remedies using herbs, minerals and animal parts • Bleeding and purging to restore the balance of the humours (Galen's Theory of Opposites) • Rest, exercise and diet
Surgery	• Simple surgery on visible tumours and wounds; splints for fractured bones • Plants such as opium dulled pain but there were no effective anaesthetics • Wine, vinegar or honey used to clean wounds but could not prevent infections • Sewed up large wounds or used cauterisation to stop heavy bleeding
Public health and prevention	• Kings and governments not expected to improve public health • Epidemic diseases and plagues could not be stopped • Towns employed rakers and made laws but struggled to keep streets clean • Animal and human waste in streets; open sewers; lack of clean water
Hospitals and healers	• Mothers and family members treated most illnesses • Physicians were trained at university but only treated the rich

Review 2

Factors

For the big 16-mark question in the exam, you need to explain the role played by factors in the development of medicine. Factors can help medicine progress but they can also hinder it.

Look at the example paragraph below. It explains how religion **hindered** the development of medicine. Note how the highlighted connective 'this meant that' helps to develop the answer – proving that this factor played an important role.

1. Complete this first paragraph, making sure you explain how religious beliefs also discouraged people during the Middle Ages from challenging Galen and developing new ideas.
2. Then, write a second paragraph in which you explain how Christianity did contribute positively to medical progress and treatments. For example, you could explore how Christianity encouraged the establishment of hospitals.

> Religion played an important role in influencing medicine and public health in the medieval period. Epidemics such as the Black Death were seen as a punishment from God. This meant that people did not look for scientific explanations of disease and did not make the link between illness and dirty water, ineffective sewers, dirty streets and overcrowded living conditions. Religious beliefs also discouraged people at the time from challenging Galen. This was because …
>
> However, the influence of religion also improved some areas of medicine. For example, …

Summarise

1. On page 17 we used the memory aid similar to the one of the right to help remember four things that medieval people believed caused disease. Can you remember all four, just by looking at the image?
2. Look at the pictures below. What four common treatments do they show from the medieval period?

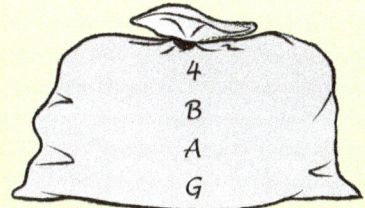

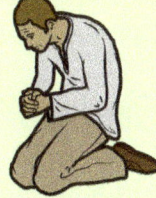 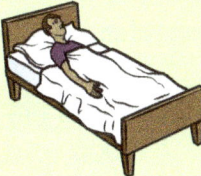 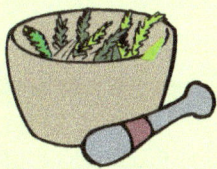 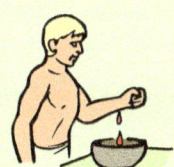

3. Draw and label your own pictures to summarise the key features of public health in towns in medieval Britain.

Period introduction: The Renaissance period, c1500–1800

4.1 Introducing ... Andreas Vesalius

Reflect

How did a Belgian studying in Italy influence medicine in Britain?

Complete your own table like the one below to record Vesalius' impact.

Area of medicine	Impact?	Explanation (say whether his work had impact in the short term or the long term)
Knowledge of the cause of disease	No	
Knowledge of the body	Yes	Short term: Vesalius' book quickly improved knowledge about anatomy around Europe.
Treatments		
Surgery		
Medical training		
Public health		

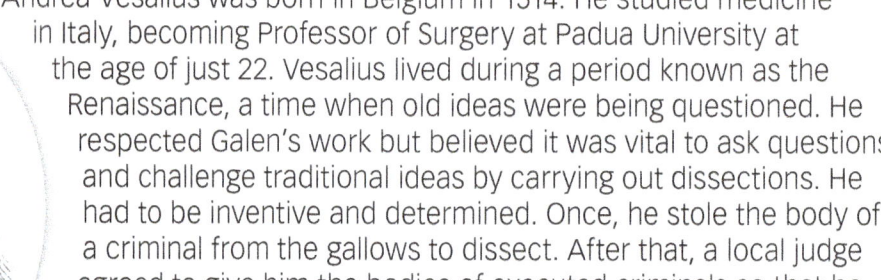

Andrea Vesalius was born in Belgium in 1514. He studied medicine in Italy, becoming Professor of Surgery at Padua University at the age of just 22. Vesalius lived during a period known as the Renaissance, a time when old ideas were being questioned. He respected Galen's work but believed it was vital to ask questions and challenge traditional ideas by carrying out dissections. He had to be inventive and determined. Once, he stole the body of a criminal from the gallows to dissect. After that, a local judge agreed to give him the bodies of executed criminals so that he could study the structure of the body more closely.

Vesalius published his work in *The Fabric of the Human Body* in 1543. He proved that Galen had made some mistakes:

- the human jaw bone is made from one bone, not two as Galen said
- the breastbone has three parts, not seven as Galen said
- blood does not flow into the heart through invisible holes in the septum – such holes do not exist.

Vesalius' book was full of illustrations showing the body in far more detail and more accurately than had ever been done before. The invention of the printing press meant the book was widely available to doctors all over Europe. By the 1560s, it was being used in England to train doctors and correct mistakes in older medical books.

His book also encouraged doctors to carry out their own dissections. The first dissection, by an anatomist in Cambridge, was carried out in 1565. However, many doctors stuck to traditional ideas, not daring to think for themselves, still saying it was wrong to challenge Galen. Vesalius faced lots of criticism and was forced to leave Padua University.

The significance of Vesalius

Before Vesalius – the story so far

In the Middle Ages:
- medical training was based on books written by Galen
- the study of anatomy had almost disappeared; doctors were taught that Galen had given a fully correct description of anatomy so there was no point trying to find things out for themselves
- dissection was carried out to show that Galen was right, not to challenge him.

Vesalius' key ideas/key findings

- **Knowledge**: Correcting mistakes made by Galen.
- **Attitudes**: The importance of dissection and asking questions.

Short-term impact (the next 30 years)

- Vesalius' book quickly improved knowledge about anatomy around Europe.
- It helped change attitudes. Some doctors realised there was more to be learned.
- It helped change training. Some doctors carried out human (not animal) dissection to learn more.
- It triggered other research into anatomy. Using the approach outlined by Vesalius, one of his students (Falloppio) published a book showing the structure of the human skull and ear.

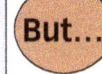

LIMITATIONS

- No one was healthier as a result of Vesalius' work.
- He did not affect understanding of disease or treatments. For most of the period 1500–c1700, doctors still based their treatments on Galen and other ancient writers.
- Even in 1668, Samuel Pepys noted in his diary that the leading expert on eye problems in London had only ever seen animals' eyes dissected, never a human eye.

Long-term impact (the next 300 years)

- Gradually, other doctors followed Vesalius' example and started to challenge traditional ideas in other areas of medicine. Later in the sixteenth century, Ambroise Paré developed new surgical techniques. In the seventeenth century, William Harvey proved – through dissection and experiments – how blood is circulated around the body by the heart.
- Vesalius' insistence on enquiry was a turning point. By the late 1600s, most students were encouraged to find things out themselves and gain hands-on experience of dissections.

Revision Tip

A good memory aid summarises the key points in as few words as possible and has a mnemonic or a drawing to help trigger memory.

A = Anatomy (the main area of medicine that Vesalius worked in)

B = Book (*The Fabric of the Human Body* spread this knowledge)

C = Challenged (traditional ideas – particularly Galen)

D = Dissection (showed the importance of dissecting human bodies)

E = Education (doctors should learn by finding out things for themselves – rather than just by reading books)

The ABCDE of Vesalius

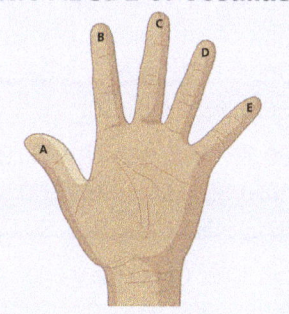

Topic 4: The impact of the Renaissance on Britain

4.2 How knowledge of anatomy improved

Research & Record

What factors helped change ideas about anatomy?
Complete the table below using the information on this page and on pages 30–31.

Think carefully about the language you use to state how important each factor was. In column 2, choose a word or phrase from the scale on the right to show the level of importance. Do not fill in column 3 if you think a factor had no or only minimal impact.

Essential	No change could have happened without it
Important	Without it change might have been less widespread or significant
Minimal	Had only a little impact
No importance	No influence at all

Factor	Importance in new ideas about anatomy	Explanation
Religion	Important	During the Renaissance, people began to challenge traditional ideas.
Individual genius	Essential	Vesalius …
Chance		
Communication		
Government		
Warfare		
Science & technology		

Printing

For centuries, books had been copied out by hand. In 1436, Johannes Gutenberg worked out a better and cheaper way to produce books – the printing press. His invention created a printing revolution. By 1500, printing presses were common throughout western Europe.

One advantage of printing was that each copy was the same. This had not happened in books copied by hand, where errors could creep in because of the hand-copying process.

Some printed books were highly illustrated such as Source 1 from Andreas Vesalius' book on anatomy. In Italy, many artists were interested in dissection and Vesalius used their artwork to illustrate his book. Thousands of copies of Vesalius' book were sold all over Europe. As a result, doctors in Britain improved their knowledge of anatomy.

Enquiry

Printing also helped spread Greek and Roman ideas. Nearly 600 printed editions of Galen's books were produced. Surprisingly, instead of continuing Galen's ideas, they helped to encourage people to think and to challenge them.

People even saw that Galen himself loved enquiry. He asked questions, challenged old ideas and suggested new ones. If it was OK for Galen and the Greeks to do this, so could the people of the Renaissance!

This spirit of enquiry changed the way that doctors were trained. It also helped lead to a scientific revolution in the late seventeenth and eighteenth centuries when new discoveries were made and old ideas challenged.

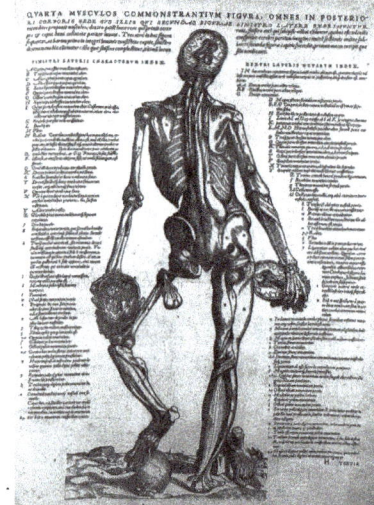

▲ **SOURCE 1** Page from *The Fabric of the Human Body*, published in 1543

Apply ▶ Exam Practice

How useful is Source A to a historian studying how traditional ideas about medicine were challenged during the Renaissance? (8 marks)

Students crowd around the body so they can see what Vesalius is doing rather than simply listening to Galen being read out.

Vesalius is in the centre, dissecting the body himself.

Galen and other Greek doctors are shown at the same level as Vesalius, not higher up as if superior.

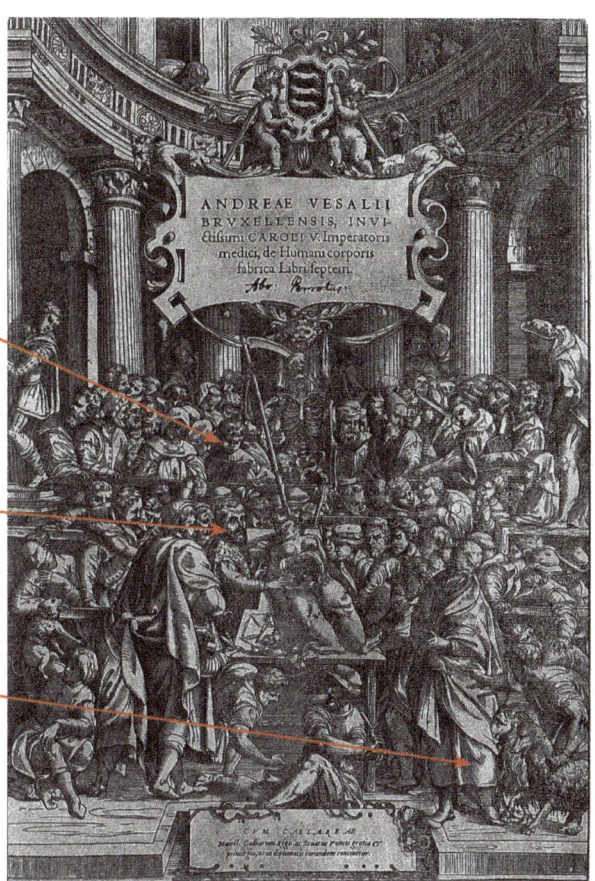

▶ **SOURCE A** The title page of Vesalius' *The Fabric of the Human Body*. This book was published in 1543 and contained a detailed and fully illustrated description of human anatomy

Exam Tip

Question 1 style: How useful is source …?

Your exam will start with a source-based question.

- You have to analyse the source carefully, identifying what it tells you and explaining why it is useful.
- You should focus on how it is useful. The examiner does not want you to highlight problems with it.
- You have about 10 minutes to answer this question in the exam. Two paragraphs would be enough for a high-level answer. You should aim to make two main points about why the source is useful. Begin each paragraph with your main point. For example,

Source A is useful because it shows how Vesalius challenged traditional ideas about how medical students should be taught …

Furthermore, the source shows how attitudes towards Galen were being challenged …

In the rest of the paragraphs, develop and support your main points by referring to the content, provenance and your wider knowledge.

C The content of the source

Before you begin to write, annotate the key features of the source, as we have in the example above.

P The provenance of the source

Remember that Vesalius supervised the engravings of the illustrations in his book personally. He would have thought very carefully about the image he wanted to go on the title page. The source, therefore, gives us an excellent insight into the key messages that Vesalius wanted to get across about approaches to anatomy, training and dissection.

K Your own knowledge of the period

You will need to bring in your own knowledge to explain how the title page of Vesalius' book shows how he challenged traditional ideas. Remember that:

- Before Vesalius, professors sat and read Galen aloud, while demonstrators did the dissection.
- Vesalius believed that it was vital to ask questions and challenge traditional ideas by carrying out dissections. The title page of his book, *The Fabric of the Human Body*, tells us a lot about his attitudes towards anatomy and teaching medical students.

4.3 The work of William Harvey

Research & Record

Why was the work of William Harvey so significant?

Read page 34 and gather evidence to support the arguments in the table. You will be able to use these notes to answer the exam question on page 35.

Argument	Support
In the short term, Harvey showed that Galen was wrong about blood being manufactured in the liver.	Harvey challenged these ideas by showing …
In the longer term, Harvey's methods set a strong example to future doctors investigating physiology.	For example, later in the 1600s, Malphigi …

How did William Harvey change physiology?

William Harvey was born in 1578 and studied medicine in Cambridge and in Padua (Italy, the same place as Vesalius!) He later became doctor to King Charles I.

Through dissection, detailed observation and scientific experiment, Harvey developed new ideas about physiology (the way the human body works). In 1628, Harvey published his 'An Anatomical Account of the Motion of the Heart and Blood'. During the medieval period, the Arab doctor, Ibn-al-Nafis had put forward the idea that blood circulates around the body (see page 21). However, Harvey was the first to prove this theory.

Through experiments, he showed that:

- The heart pumps blood around the body. Harvey worked out that the amount of blood going into the arteries each hour was three times the weight of a man. This showed that the same blood must be being pumped around the body by the heart.
- The body has a one-way system for the blood. He tried to pump liquid past the valves in the veins but could not do so. Harvey used finger pressure demonstrations that showed that valves in veins always directed blood towards the heart.

How did future generations build on Harvey's work?

Short term

Harvey's discovery was only gradually accepted. Some doctors ignored his theory. Others said that he was wrong because he was challenging Galen. It was nearly 50 years before the teachers at the University of Paris taught Harvey's ideas rather than Galen's. Harvey himself said that after he published his discovery, fewer patients came to see him. Many thought his idea mad.

Longer term

However, in the longer term, Harvey's ideas were accepted and they mark a turning point in the history of medicine. Many areas of medicine today (such as heart surgery or injections) depend on precise understanding of how blood circulates and how the heart works. Harvey's theories also explained for the first time how poisons could spread so rapidly through the body.

Harvey could not explain everything about the circulation of the blood. He did not know how blood moves from the arteries to the veins, but other doctors followed Harvey's scientific methods to build on his work. Professor Marcello Malphigi used one of the first effective **microscopes** to discover the tiny blood vessels, known as capillaries, which carry blood from arteries to veins.

The work of Vesalius and Harvey led to a scientific revolution in the late seventeenth and eighteenth centuries. In 1660, the Royal Society was established. Members of the society met weekly to discuss ideas and carry out experiments (see page 45).

Exam Tip – Question 2: How to prove significance

Think before you write using the '4Ds'

Decode – work out the focus of the question.

Staying focused on the question is crucial. Including information that is not relevant or writing about the wrong topic wastes time and gains no marks. Here's how to 'decode' a question.

What are the command words? The question asks you to 'Explain'. You need to do more than describe, you have to **analyse**.

What is the conceptual focus? The concept is **significance**, which means what changed because of Harvey's work. So, you need to say briefly what medicine was like before Harvey's discoveries. Then explain how Harvey challenged traditional ideas about physiology. The table you have just produced should help you.

Link Harvey's work with changes that took place in later generations. Aim to explain two or three changes that took place.

Apply ▶ Exam Practice

Question 2 style: Explain the significance

Use your research from page 34 and the guidance on the opposite page to answer the exam question below.

Explain the significance of the work of William Harvey in the development of medicine. **(8 marks)**

What is the content focus? It's about the work of William Harvey but do not simply describe what he did. The focus of this question is on how this work helped medicine **develop**. This means covering the long-term as well as the short-term importance of his work.

How many marks are available? 8 marks indicates you should spend about 10 minutes on the question and write a couple of paragraphs.

Decide how to organise your answer before you start to write.

You do not have the time to tell the story of Harvey's life. The focus is on the impact of his work. Decide the main points you want to make and then organise these points into two paragraphs. One possible approach is:

Paragraph 1: Short-term impact – explain how Harvey challenged Galen's ideas through careful experimentation and dissection.

Paragraph 2: Long-term impact – explain how others built on Harvey's work and why it was an important breakthrough.

Develop your answer – make sure you explain and support the points you make.

Do not simply state that Harvey challenged Galen – explain how and give specific examples.

Do not simply state that Harvey's discoveries were important for many areas of medicine. Explain why they were so important and give examples of how his work is relevant to medicine today.

Demonstrate complex thinking.

Complex thinking earns the top marks in this exam. For example:
- **How fast did change occur?** Do not give the impression that change was instant. Were Harvey's ideas accepted immediately or did the significance of his work take time to be accepted?

4.4 The work of Ambroise Paré

Research & Record

How did Paré change surgery?

Using pages 36 and 37, fill in the table below to show how Paré changed surgery and the factors that helped him introduce new surgical techniques.

	Surgery in the medieval period	Changes introduced by Paré	What factors helped?
Helping amputees	Amputees used crutches.	Paré developed artificial limbs	Individual genius – Paré Better technology
Preventing infection	Gunpowder was thought to be poisonous, so wounds were treated with boiling oil to kill the poison.	Paré …	Chance …
Stopping blood loss	Wounds and amputations were closed by cauterisation (putting a red-hot iron onto the wound to seal the blood vessels).		

How did Paré's experiences on the battlefield help him?

Ambroise Paré was born in France, in 1510. He learned his surgical skills as an apprentice to his brother, who was a barber-surgeon. From 1536, he spent 20 years as an army surgeon. His experiences on the battlefield led to important breakthroughs in surgery.

Artificial limbs

Paré designed and arranged the making of false limbs for wounded soldiers. He designed more than 50 kinds of false body parts. He included drawings of them in his books to spread the idea. Skilled armourers (makers of armour and weapons) made the false limbs. The best even allowed the user to hold a sword and fight.

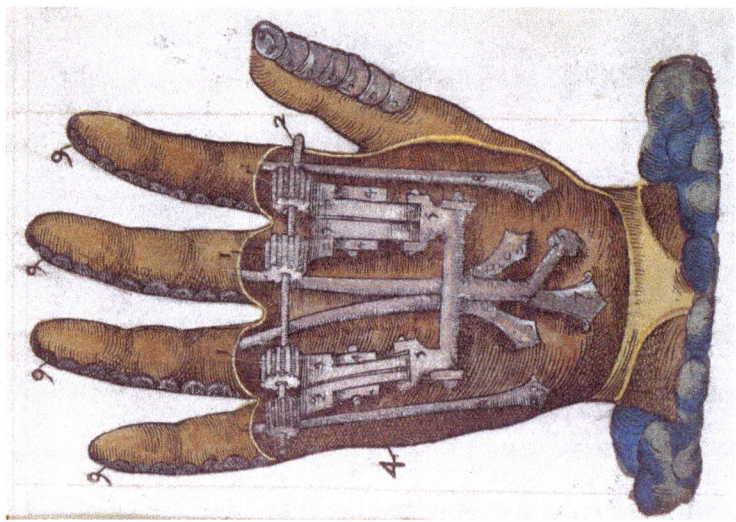

▶ **SOURCE 1** This wood engraving, showing the mechanism inside a false hand, appeared in one of Paré's books published in 1564

Dealing with gunshot wounds

Like other surgeons at the time, Paré thought that the only way to stop wounds becoming poisoned by gunpowder was to pour on boiling oil. As you can imagine, this was extremely painful for the patient!

However, on one occasion Paré ran out of oil. Instead, he mixed up an ointment or lotion made from egg yolks, oil of roses and turpentine. That night he struggled to sleep, fearing that he would awake to find his patients dead or poisoned. To his surprise, the next morning, he found that the patients he had treated with the ointment were in little pain and that their wounds were not inflamed or infected. In contrast, the soldiers on whom he had used the boiling oil were in a great deal of pain and had swelling around their wounds.

Paré's work became widely known through his books, which were translated into other languages, including English. His new method of using ointments rather than boiling oil became widely accepted.

Ligatures

Paré knew that cauterisation was extremely painful and did not always stop bleeding. Instead of cauterising, he experimented with tying **ligatures** (silk threads) around individual blood vessels to stop bleeding. This was slower than cauterising, for example, 53 ligatures had to be tied when a leg was amputated at the thigh. Ligatures were also dangerous because the thread could carry infection. It was not until effective antiseptics were developed 300 years later that ligatures could be used without the risk of infection.

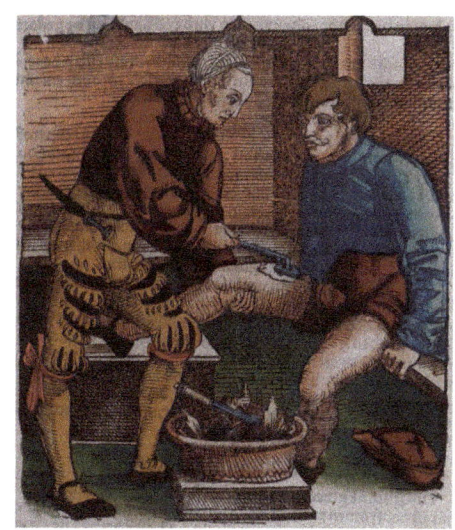

▶ **SOURCE 2** A wound being cauterised. In reality, the patient would have been struggling and screaming with pain. This wood engraving dates from around the fifteenth–sixteenth century

Paré's impact on surgery

Paré's books were widely read and his techniques were adopted by surgeons across Europe. Paré went on to become the most famous surgeon in Europe, serving as the surgeon to the kings of France. He affected:

- **Attitudes**: Paré encouraged surgeons to think for themselves and try out new techniques. He showed that improvements were possible. In England, surgeons followed his approach and experimented with new ideas. Elizabeth I's surgeon, William Clowes, agreed with Paré and produced a book showing how to deal with battlefield wounds.
- **Status**: Paré helped to raise the status of barber-surgeons. In England, Henry VIII gave barber-surgeons a charter to form the Company of Barber-Surgeons, making it a respected profession.

However, Paré's discoveries did not help surgeons overcome the major problems they faced. Thanks to Paré, some surgical treatments were less painful but:

- Surgeons still did not have access to effective anaesthetics.
- They had no effective antiseptics to stop infection.
- They did not understand about blood groups or have fast ways of stopping major bleeding.

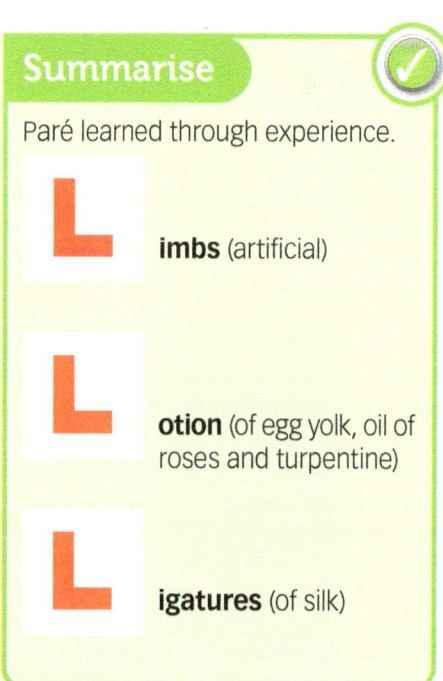

Summarise

Paré learned through experience.

L imbs (artificial)

L otion (of egg yolk, oil of roses and turpentine)

L igatures (of silk)

Topic 5: Dealing with disease

5.1 Traditional and new methods of treating illness

Research & Record

How far did everyday treatments change?

1. As you read through pages 38 and 39, use a table like this to record how the Renaissance period saw a mixture of old and new forms of treatment.
2. Then evaluate how much change this period saw in the treatment of illnesses. Choose the appropriate phrase from the scale below and explain why you have come to this conclusion.
3. Choose the strongest piece of evidence to support your overall conclusion.

Evidence of continuity in medical treatments	Evidence of changes in medical treatments

a **total change** in the way that illness was treated	**significant changes**	some changes but **mainly continuity**	**considerable continuity**	**no changes** in the way that illness was treated

Bleeding and purging

During the Renaissance, bleeding was still one of the most common treatments. Physicians continued to believe that many illnesses were caused when the humours in the patient's body were out of balance. Bleeding and purging were meant to correct the balance, even though this must have weakened the patient.

▼ **SOURCE 1** This painting by a Dutch artist shows a physician binding up a woman's arm after blood-letting. It was painted in 1666. You can see the bleeding cup on the table

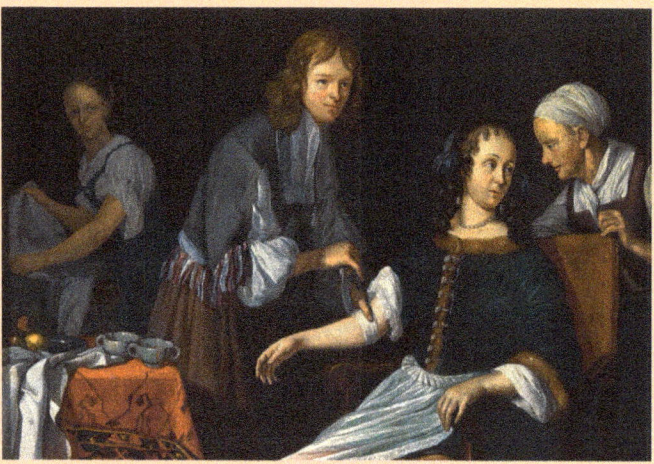

Herbal remedies

Home remedies were handed down through generations from mother to daughter. They used everyday ingredients such as honey, which we now know helps fight infection.

The printing revolution meant that more people learned to read and could buy 'herbals' (books with advice on herbal remedies). One of the most popular books was *The Complete Herbal* by Nicholas Culpepper, which described the properties of herbs that could be used at home and which parts of the body or which ailments they were good for. Culpepper also linked each herb to one of the signs of the zodiac or one of the planets.

New treatments from abroad

European explorers brought back new treatments. For example:

- Rhubarb from Asia was widely used to purge the bowels.
- The bark of the cinchona tree from South America was used to treat fevers. In Europe, it became known as **quinine** and helped many who had malaria.
- Less helpfully, opium from Turkey was used as an anaesthetic. It worked, but it was highly addictive and easy to overdose!
- Tobacco was greeted as a **'cure-all'** when it arrived from America, being recommended for toothache, poisoned wounds, joint pains and as protection from plague. One schoolboy commented that during the Plague of 1665, he was beaten for 'not smoking often enough'!

Quackery

Quackery had begun in the Middle Ages. **Quacks** were travelling salesmen. They had no medical qualifications. They travelled from town to town selling their medicines and pills, which they claimed could cure anything.

- During the Renaissance period, quackery boomed. Men like Joshua Ward made a lot of money by selling pills that they claimed could cure every illness, including gout, scurvy and syphilis. All the pills did was make people sweat a lot!
- Later in the period, James Morrison made his fortune selling his 'Vegetable Pills', encouraging people to take as many as possible to stay healthy. The pills contained mainly purgatives and caused numerous deaths due to excessive bowel movements.

Treatments based on superstition

▼ **SOURCE 2** This engraving shows people being touched by Charles II. Between 1660 and 1682, over 92,000 people visited the King, believing that if he touched them they would be cured from scrofula, a skin disease known as the 'King's Evil'

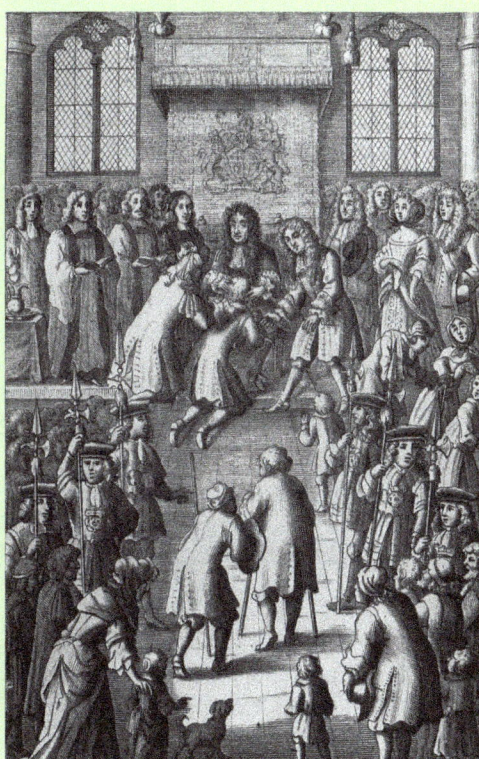

▼ **SOURCE 3** From *The New London Dispensary*, 1682

To cure malaria, take the hair and nails of the patient, cut them small and either give them to the birds in a roasted egg or put them in a hole in an oak tree or a plane tree. Stop up the hole with a peg of the same tree.

The bezoar stone – testing a magical cure

This is a story that shows how superstitious ideas still existed but were being challenged.

In 1566, a visitor to King Charles of France gave the King a **bezoar stone** from the stomach of a goat. The visitor said it would cure all poisons. The King's surgeon (Ambroise Paré, whom you already know about) told him it could not possibly do so because a hot poison needed a cold antidote and vice-versa.

Paré then suggested they test the stone. A man who had been sentenced to death for theft was offered the chance to live if he took poison and then the bezoar stone. If the bezoar stone worked, he would be free! The man accepted the chance, took poison and then the stone. He died in agony several hours later. It was another triumph for experiment, though not so good for the thief!

5.2 Case study: The Great Plague of 1665

Reflect

How far were responses to the 1665 Plague similar to the Black Death?

In the exam, Question 2 tests your ability to compare two events or developments from different time periods. This activity will help you practise comparison.

1. How much can you remember about the Black Death? Try to fill in the second column of a table like this from memory alone.
2. Check what you have done against your research notes and pages 26 and 27 in this book. Fill in any gaps and correct any errors.
3. Use these two pages to fill in the third column.
4. Reflect on what you have found out:
   - What are the two strongest similarities?
   - Why were responses to the two events so similar?

	Black Death, 1348–49	The Plague, 1665
Causes		
Beliefs – what did people believe caused it?		
Treatments		
Methods of prevention		
Consequences – short- and long-term impact		

Causes: What was the Plague of 1665?

After the Black Death of 1348, plague never completely disappeared. For example, in 1604, 30 per cent of the people of York died from plague. Outbreaks like this happened all over the country.

Then, in 1665, another outbreak of bubonic plague killed around 100,000 people in London and many thousands more all over Britain. One major reason was that London was so overcrowded and full of dirt – which encouraged rats.

Explanations: What did people think caused it?

Many people still believed that God had sent plague to punish them for their sins. The government ordered days of public prayer and fasting so that people could publicly confess their sins and beg God to be merciful.

Others blamed the movements of planets or poisonous air, just as in the fourteenth century. If you look closely at the plague doctor's clothes and equipment, you can work out what people thought caused the plague.

- The doctor is wearing a hat, very thick clothes, gloves and boots to avoid direct contact with those who had the plague or their belongings.
- The nose cone is full of sweet-smelling herbs to ward off bad air.
- An **amulet** (jewellery) to ward off evil spirits is hidden under the sleeve of the coat.

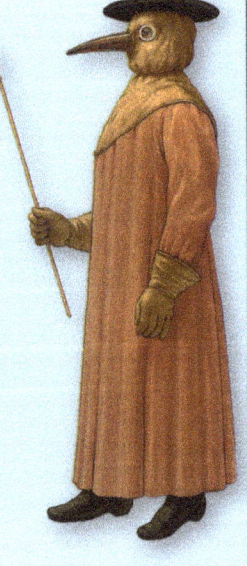

Treatments: How did people try to treat the plague?

- Doctors still had no cures for the plague. Physicians might have recommended bleeding or purging, but most physicians left London to save themselves from plague.
- People prayed for sick people, or gave them magical or religious charms to wear.
- They cut open the buboes to let the pus out.
- Quacks sold 'Great Medicines' which they claimed had saved 'vast numbers' of lives. One such medicine, Theriac, or London Treacle, contained wine, herbs, spices, honey and opium.
- There were many different herbal remedies proposed. Some were a mixture of herbs and superstition. For example: *Wrap in woollen clothes, make the sick person sweat, which if he do, keep warm until the sores begin to rise. Then apply to the sores live pigeons cut in half or else a plaster made of yolk of an egg, honey, herb of grace and wheat flour.*

Prevention: How did people try to prevent it from spreading?

People believed it was vital to keep the air sweet to ward off the bad air. They hung bunches of strong-smelling herbs (such as lavender or sage) in doorways and windows. They even carried bundles of herbs under their noses as they walked through the streets.

The Mayor of London did his best to stop the plague spreading from infected houses.

- Those who had the disease were shut up in their homes and watchmen stood guard to stop anyone going in or out.
- When anyone died, the body was examined by 'women searchers' to check that plague was the cause.
- Bedding had to be hung in the smoke of fires before it was used again.
- Fires were lit in the streets to cleanse the air of poisons.

Other regulations showed that people were making a connection between dirt and disease, even if they could not explain the link scientifically.

- Householders were ordered to sweep the street outside their doors.
- Pigs, dogs and cats were not to be kept inside the city. Stray dogs and cats were killed.
- Plays, bear-baitings and games were banned to prevent the assembly of large crowds.

However, these measures did not really work because:

- Parliament refused to turn the orders into laws because MPs refused to be shut in their houses.
- The King and his council left London. They discussed what to do about plague three times in seven months, but two of those discussions were about the King's safety.
- Nine men were put in charge of dealing with plague in London. Six of them left London as soon as they could.
- Plague symptoms were not reported. In fact, over 20 watchmen were murdered by people escaping from houses that had been shut up.
- Not enough men could be found to work as watchmen.
- Some watchmen and women searchers took the chance to steal from sick people.

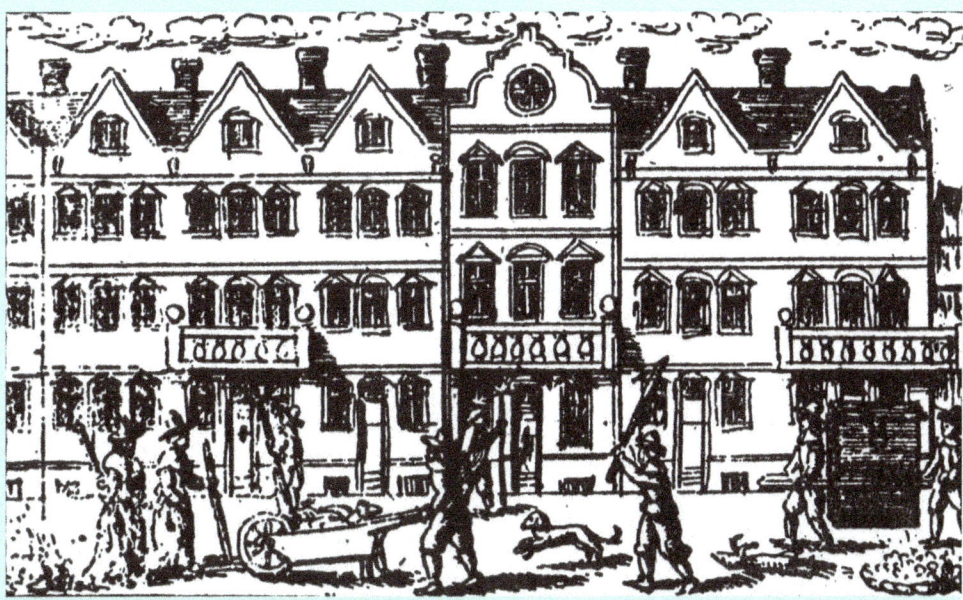

▼ **SOURCE 1** A seventeenth-century print of a London street during the plague. It shows some of the plague orders being implemented. How many can you spot?

Impact: The consequences of the Plague

The methods introduced in London by the Lord Mayor helped a little, but over a quarter of the population of London died in the Great Plague of 1665.

It took a combination of cold weather and then the Great Fire of London in 1666 to put an end to the Great Plague.

Following the Great Fire, central London was completely rebuilt. Narrow streets and wooden buildings were replaced by stone and brick buildings, and wider, better-paved streets.

For a time, London was healthier, but as the city became more and more crowded again during the Industrial Revolution, the benefits of the rebuilding disappeared.

5.3 The growth of hospitals

Research & Record

How far did hospitals change in the period 1500–1800?

Complete a table like this using the information on this page and on page 43.

Key questions	Medieval hospitals	Hospitals 1500–1800	Evaluation/Extent of change
Organisation Who set up and ran the hospitals?	The Church – monasteries	Charities and some local councils	Significant change but still not organised by the national government
Staffing Who provided the medical care?	Not physicians Mainly nuns		
Patients Who did they treat?	Mainly people living in poverty and older people – rarely sick people in case they spread disease		
Treatments How were these patients treated?	Mainly prayer, rest and food Some herbal remedies		
Scale How many hospitals were there? How large were they?	500 (by 1400) Mainly small with 5 or 6 beds		

Many medieval hospitals were part of monasteries so they closed when Henry VIII closed the monasteries in the 1530s. However, some were taken over by town councils, especially the alms-houses that looked after older people living in poverty.

In London, the city council and charity helped to keep St Bartholomew's Hospital open. By the 1660s, it had 12 wards and up to 300 patients, looked after by 3 physicians and 3 surgeons, 15 nursing sisters and a larger number of nursing helpers.

Nursing sisters treated patients with herbal remedies but nursing helpers did the heavy, manual work – washing, cleaning and preparing food. They had no medical training.

During the eighteenth century, things began to change. More hospitals were established, including specialist hospitals (such as maternity hospitals).

By 1800, London's hospitals were treating more than 20,000 patients a year. Most large towns had a hospital.

However:

- Hospitals treated relatively minor complaints (like bronchitis or leg ulcers).
- People with infectious diseases were still not admitted. Most provided just food, warmth and prayer.
- The types of treatment available were still based around the four humours. Bleeding and purging were common.
- Anyone with any money preferred to pay for a doctor or nurse to look after them at home.
- By 1700, London's population had risen to over half a million people, yet it only had two large medical hospitals.

Exam Tip – Question 3: 'comparison' questions

Look at the two exam questions below. Use your research notes and the advice on this page to answer both questions. The first question has been started for you at the bottom of the page.

Explain two ways in which hospitals in the 1400s and hospitals in the 1700s were similar. Explain your answer with reference to both time periods. (8 marks)	Step 1: Identify the **content focus** of the question	**Explain two ways in which the Black Death in the Middle Ages and the Great Plague of 1665 were similar. Explain your answer with reference to both time periods. (8 marks)**
This question compares **one feature** (i.e. hospitals) in two different time periods.		This question compares **two events** (i.e. Black Death and Great Plague) from different periods.
Focus on **similarities**. Do not go into differences.	Step 2: Identify the **conceptual focus** of the question	Focus on **similarities**. Do not go into differences.
When you compare **features** of medicine in different periods, you need some key questions to guide you. Try these for hospitals:	Step 3: **Plan** You will have about 10 minutes for this 8 mark question in the exam. Aim for two well-developed paragraphs. Base each paragraph around a similarity and **make direct comparisons** across the two periods. DO NOT simply describe one event/period in one paragraph and another event/period in the other!	When you compare **events** you could focus on the following questions:
1. **Importance**: How many hospitals were there? How many people did they treat? Who did they treat?		1. **Causes**: What caused the event?
2. **Healers**: Who treated patients? Were they trained?		2. **Development**: How did people respond? What did they believe caused it? How did they then try and treat or prevent the disease?
3. **Treatments**: How were patients treated? What methods of treatment were used? How effective were they?		3. **Consequences**: What were the **short-** and **long-term** consequences of the event?

Example answer

Medieval hospitals tended to care for older people and those living in poverty. They were small in scale and rarely took in people who had infectious diseases. **This continued to be the case** throughout the Renaissance period. There were some exceptions, like St Bartholomew's in London, but most hospitals **still did not** admit people with infectious diseases. Anyone with any money paid for a doctor or nurse to look after them at home. **In both periods**, the government did not take responsibility for funding and organising hospitals. During the Middle Ages, hospitals were set up by the Church and local charities. During the Renaissance period, local charities and councils **continued to play an important role** in setting up hospitals or taking over hospitals such as St Bartholomew's that had been run by the Church.

There were **also similarities in terms of** how patients were treated. In hospitals in the Middle Ages …

5.4 Changes to the training and status of surgeons and physicians

Research & Record

Who treated sick people between 1500 and 1800 and how well trained were they?

The Renaissance period saw changes. However, change was slow and there was also continuity in who treated sick people and how they were trained.

Use pages 44 and 45 to find examples to place on the set of scales (right).

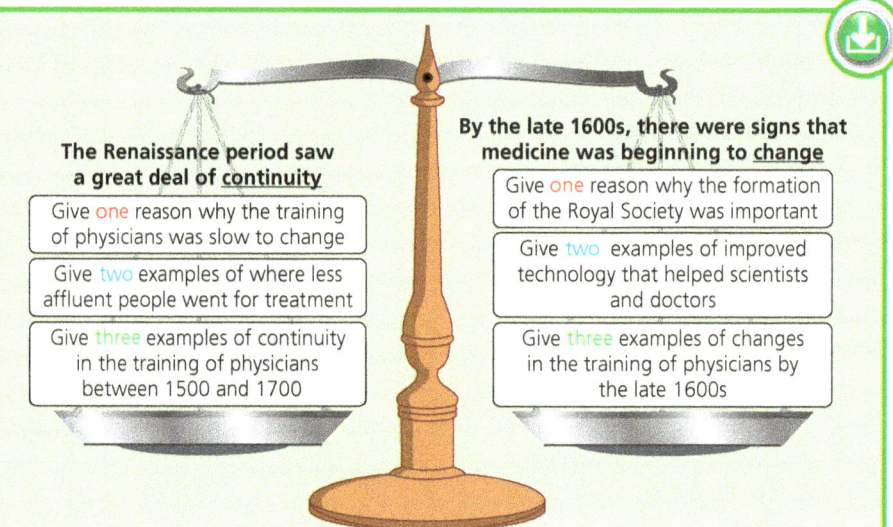

The Renaissance period saw a great deal of continuity
- Give one reason why the training of physicians was slow to change
- Give two examples of where less affluent people went for treatment
- Give three examples of continuity in the training of physicians between 1500 and 1700

By the late 1600s, there were signs that medicine was beginning to change
- Give one reason why the formation of the Royal Society was important
- Give two examples of improved technology that helped scientists and doctors
- Give three examples of changes in the training of physicians by the late 1600s

Training and technology

Through the 1500s and 1600s, most university-trained physicians still accepted Hippocrates' theory that illness was caused by an imbalance in the body's humours. Their training still concentrated on the writings of Greek doctors, especially Galen, and Arab doctors such as Ibn Sina.

Many physicians also read the work of Vesalius, Paré and Harvey, but were still reluctant to accept that Galen could have been wrong.

However, by the late 1600s, the training of doctors was finally beginning to change:

- In a few hospitals (for example, Edinburgh in Scotland and St Bartholomew's in London) part of a physician's training took place on the wards.
- Training emphasised the importance of a scientific approach, observing symptoms and trying out treatments.
- More doctors did dissections.
- They were helped by improved technology. Medical equipment was beginning to improve, for example, better microscopes and the first thermometers.

Who did most people go to for treatment?

Although physicians were highly regarded and better trained, most people still could not afford physicians so continued to prefer more familiar and cheaper remedies from surgeons and apothecaries (who prepared medical remedies from the drugs stored in their shops – as a pharmacist might today).

The first person to treat nearly all illness was the wife or mother of the sick person, or the local wise woman, skilled in herbal remedies. Travelling quacks were also popular.

The influence of the Royal Society

In 1645, a group of people interested in discussing new scientific ideas got together in London. They met weekly to discuss new ideas in physics, botany, astronomy, medicine and other sciences. The Society published books and articles to spread new ideas and discoveries.

The Society built its own laboratory and bought equipment such as microscopes. They demonstrated experiments (such as the one shown in Source 1).

After seventeen years, in 1662, the group became known as the Royal Society after King Charles II attended meetings to hear talks and watch experiments. He even had a laboratory and an observatory built in one of his palaces.

This experimental approach to science changed the ways that doctors thought. They were more prepared to challenge old ideas and search for new discoveries. By the late 1600s, support for the ideas of Galen had begun to fade.

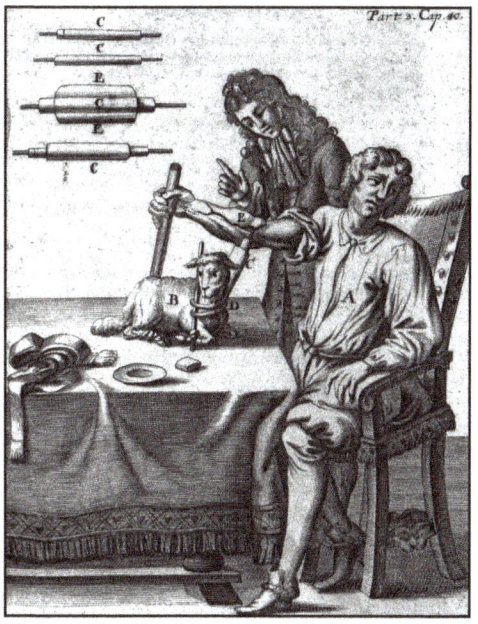

▲ **SOURCE 1** In 1665, Richard Lower, a member of the Royal Society, made the first experimental blood transfusion. He transfused blood from a dog to another dog and later from a sheep to a man

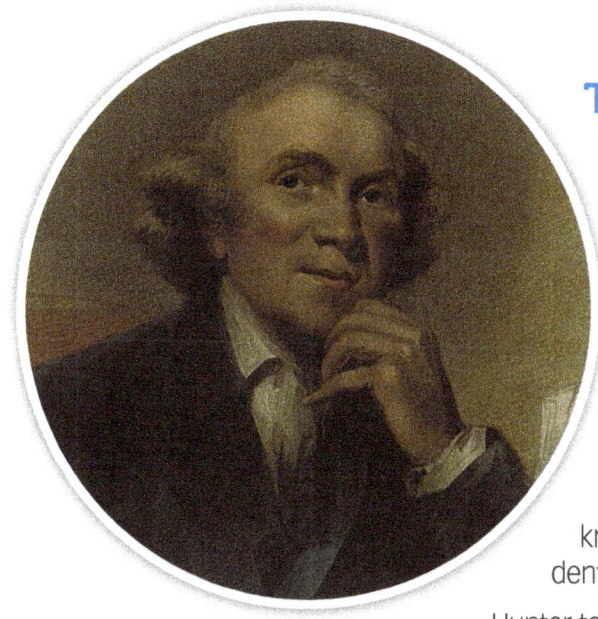

The influence of John Hunter

The training and status of surgeons began to change during the eighteenth century. John Hunter set up his own anatomy school and surgical practice. He trained hundreds of surgeons. He encouraged a scientific approach and experimentation. One individual inspired by Hunter was Edward Jenner (see pages 46 and 47), who developed a vaccination against smallpox.

Hunter was surgeon to King George III and Surgeon General to the British army. This gave him great influence. His books were widely read and helped to improve surgical knowledge. They covered a wide range of topics, including dentistry, venereal disease and how to treat gunshot wounds.

Hunter tested new techniques in surgery. In one famous case, he successfully treated a man with a tumour on his knee joint by tying off arteries to restrict the blood flow above the aneurysm. This encouraged new blood vessels to develop and bypass the damaged area. The usual treatment would have been to amputate the patient's leg. In another successful operation, Hunter cut away a tumour weighing 4 kilograms from a patient's neck.

In 1783, Hunter moved into a large house in Leicester Square (in London) where he arranged his collection of over 500 plant and animal species into a teaching museum. Hunter's fame reflects how surgery and anatomy was beginning to be seen as an important part of medicine. The company of surgeons was formed in 1745 and, in 1800, it was granted a royal charter, becoming the Royal College of Surgeons.

Topic 6: Prevention of disease

6.1 Edward Jenner and the smallpox vaccination

> **Research & Record**
>
> **Why was the work of Edward Jenner so significant?**
> To explain the significance of an individual you need to know three main things:
> 1. **The situation before** the individual made their discovery: what problems did people face?
> 2. **The impact at the time**: what changed as a result of their work in the short term?
> 3. **The long-term impact**: why was their work a turning point in medicine?
>
> Use pages 46–47 to make research notes under those three headings.

How did people try to prevent smallpox before Jenner?

In the 1700s, smallpox was as frightening as plague. It killed more children each year than any other disease and thousands of adults too. Survivors could be badly disfigured.

In China and Asia, a technique had been discovered to stop people catching smallpox. It was called **inoculation**. It involved spreading pus from a smallpox spot into a cut in the skin of a healthy person. If the person was lucky, they got only a mild dose of smallpox and did not catch it again because their body had developed a resistance to smallpox. During the eighteenth century, this method of prevention became popular in England.

However, there were dangers with inoculation:

- The person inoculated could get a severe dose of smallpox and die.
- The person inoculated could pass smallpox on to someone else.
- Most people could not afford inoculation so were not protected. Doctors could charge up to £20 per patient (£1500 in today's money).

How did Jenner make his discovery?

In the 1790s, Edward Jenner was an experienced doctor. He had studied under John Hunter, the greatest surgeon of the time (see page 45). He kept in touch with Hunter when he began work as a country doctor in Gloucestershire in the 1770s. Hunter taught his students to observe patients carefully and to test their ideas through experimentation. Jenner followed Hunter's advice to discover a new way of preventing smallpox.

Like other country doctors, Jenner knew that milkmaids who caught cowpox, a mild disease, never got smallpox. In the 1790s, Jenner decided to carry out experiments to see if he could use cowpox to prevent smallpox in other people. He carefully recorded each experiment in detail.

In one famous experiment, Jenner took cowpox pus from a sore on the hand of Sarah Nelmes, a dairy maid. Jenner inserted the matter into a healthy 8-year-old boy called James Phipps. Jenner then inoculated the young boy with smallpox matter, but no disease followed. Several months later, Jenner again inoculated the boy with smallpox matter, but still no disease followed.

What was the impact of Jenner's work at the time?

Jenner did 23 similar experiments. Then, in 1798, he felt sure enough of his method to publish his findings and show people how to use it. He called it vaccination (the Latin word for cow is *vacca*). Jenner's book also included his evidence that this really worked. In Britain, the government gave Jenner £30,000 to develop his work and vaccination became widely used. Deaths from smallpox fell quickly.

However, the government did not make vaccination compulsory until 1852, 50 years after Jenner's research. This was partly because there was opposition to Jenner's methods (see diagram). It took time to convince people that his methods were safe and effective. Also, some people did not think that laws should be passed to make vaccination compulsory because the government should not interfere in people's lives.

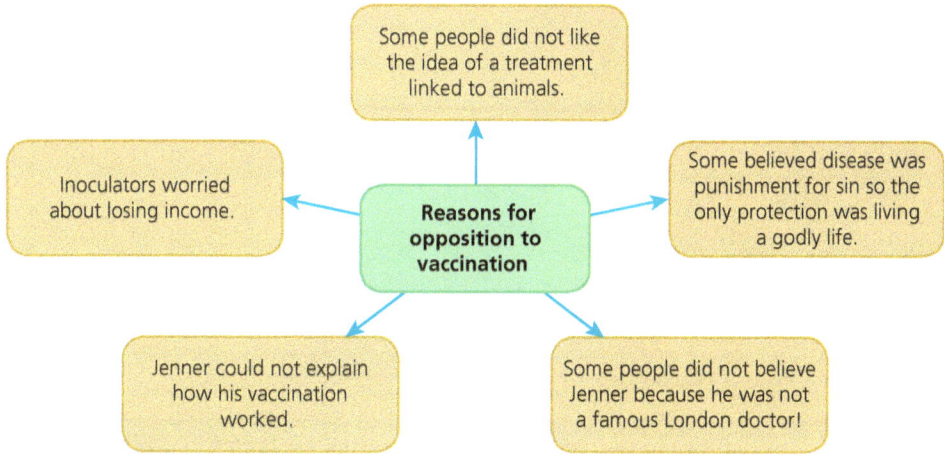

Why was Jenner's work important in the long term?

Smallpox was eradicated as a killer disease. Source 1 shows how deaths from smallpox fell in Britain. Vaccination was compulsory from 1852 but this was only strictly enforced from 1871 (after a major epidemic). Parents were fined for not having their children vaccinated. By the 1970s, smallpox had been wiped out worldwide.

Other scientists built on Jenner's work and developed vaccinations against other diseases. Jenner did not know why vaccination worked. Vaccination was a 'one-off' discovery, made because Jenner observed the connection between cowpox and smallpox. However, in the long term, after the discovery of the Germ Theory, other vaccines were developed which dramatically reduced deaths from infectious diseases (see page 50).

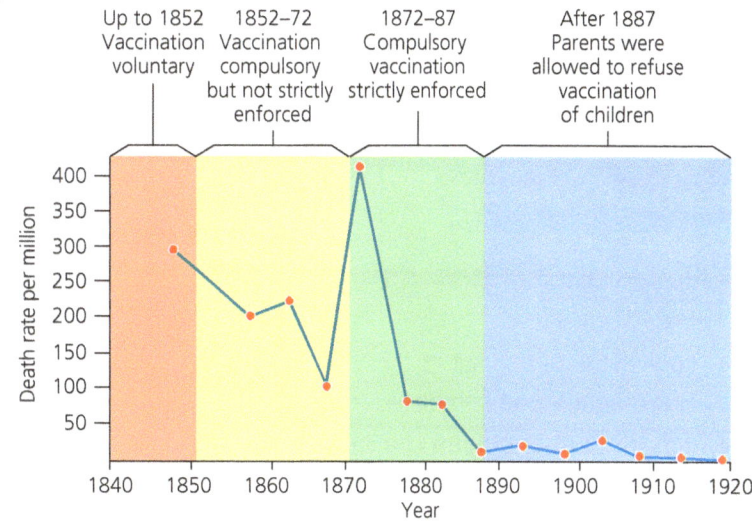

▲ **SOURCE 1** Deaths from smallpox, 1840–1920

6.2 Renaissance period review

Factor Review 1

What factors helped and hindered the development of the smallpox vaccination?

1. Source 1 shows how there was opposition to smallpox vaccinations. What factors listed in the table help to explain why there was such strong opposition?

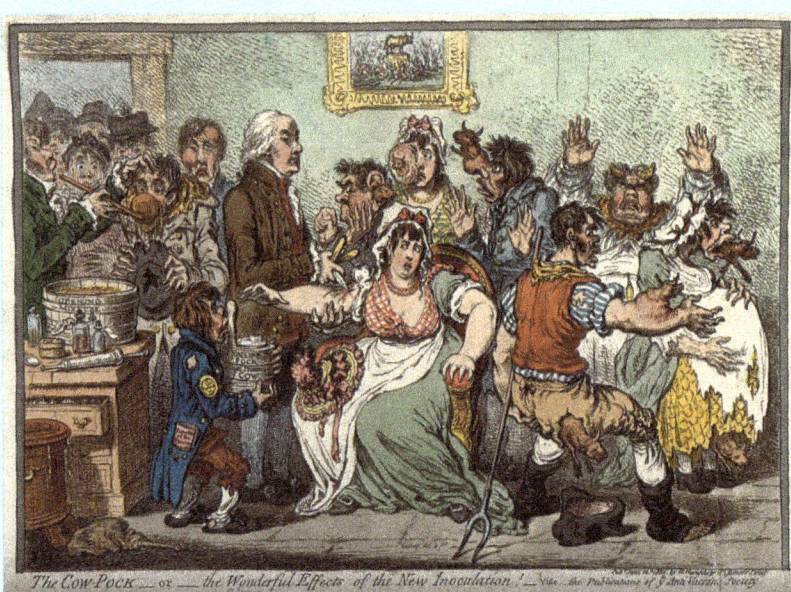

◀ **SOURCE 1** A cartoon published by the Anti-Vaccine Society in 1802. Jenner is shown vaccinating a worried woman

2. Complete a copy of the table below using pages 46–47.

Factor	How it helped	How it hindered
Government	Gave Jenner money to develop his work	Did not make vaccination compulsory straight away
The role of individuals	Jenner …	
Chance		
Communications		
Beliefs		
Science and technology		
Warfare		

Factor Review 2

What factors helped and hindered the development of medicine between 1500 and 1800?

3. Look at the period summary opposite. What factors were at work during the period?
4. Use the table you completed in part 2 to answer the questions below:

Which individual played the most important role in improving medicine in the period 1500–1800?

How far was the role played by individuals the most important factor in the development of medicine between 1500 and 1800?

Period summary c1500–1800		
Theme	Evidence of continuity	Evidence of change
Ideas about the causes of illness	• Religious beliefs still strong • Four humours • Bad air	Some people beginning to make the connection between dirt and disease (see responses to the Plague)
Knowledge of the human body and training	• Opposition to Vesalius and Harvey • Took time for ideas to be accepted	Better knowledge of: • anatomy (Vesalius) • physiology (Harvey's discovery of blood circulation)
Treatments	• Bleeding and purging • Herbal remedies • Cures still based on superstition	More herbs from overseas (e.g. quinine for malaria)
Surgery	• Cauterisation still widely used • No effective antiseptics or anaesthetics	• Improved treatment of gunshot wounds (see Paré) • Use of ligatures to stop bleeding • Artificial limbs developed
Public health and methods of prevention	Governments did little to improve public health or stop diseases from spreading	• Some attempts by the Mayor to prevent the spread of the Plague (1665) • Government funding for Jenner
Hospitals and healers	• Hospitals still did not deal with infectious diseases • Most medical care provided by women within the family or the local wise woman	• Hospitals set up by charities and local councils (e.g. St Bartholomew's in London) • Training began to change. Dissection encouraged

Summarise

Develop memory aids for the key individuals you have studied in the Renaissance period

1. Can you remember the memory aid for Vesalius? (CLUE: It should be as easy as ABC … DE). Check page 31 to see if you got it right.
2. Below is a memory aid for Jenner. Use key words and images to produce memory aids for Harvey, Paré and Hunter.

Jenner's discovery SAVED lives

S = Smallpox

A = Anti-vaccine society (opposed him)

V = Vaccination (from cowpox)

E = Experiments (e.g. James Phipps)

D = Death rates fell

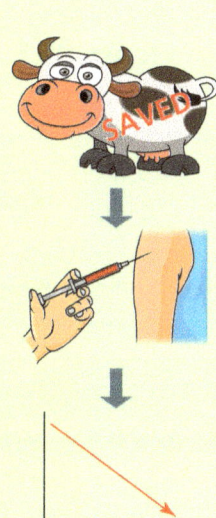

Period introduction: The nineteenth century

7.1 Introducing ... Louis Pasteur

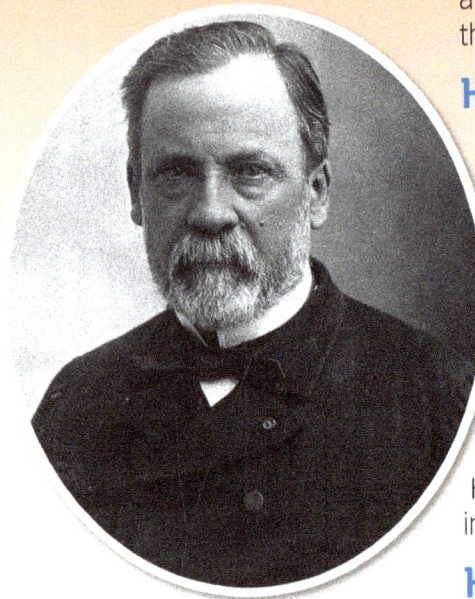

Louis Pasteur was born in France and was a university scientist, not a doctor. He was also a hugely determined man who made one of the most important breakthroughs in our understanding of disease.

How did Louis Pasteur develop the Germ Theory?

Pasteur was asked to investigate why alcoholic drinks sometimes went sour. This was costing the French beer and wine industry a lot of money. Pasteur's solution was to heat the drinks briefly to kill off disease-causing bacteria. This process became known as **pasteurisation** and was also used to stop diseases such as tuberculosis being spread through contaminated milk.

As a result of this research, Pasteur became convinced that it was germs from the air that were causing the liquids to go sour. He also speculated that, in the same way, germs might be getting into humans and perhaps be causing disease.

How did Pasteur prove that the Germ Theory was correct?

Pasteur published his 'Germ Theory' in 1861. The French government paid for Pasteur to hire research assistants and set up a new laboratory where he could carry out experiments to try to prove that his Germ Theory was correct.

In 1865, he was called in to help the silk industry. A disease was killing the silkworms. He proved that the disease was being spread by germs in the air. This was the first time it was proved that germs were causing disease in animals.

Pasteur also started to investigate human diseases. However, he struggled to identify the specific bacteria which caused individual diseases.

How did others build on Pasteur's work?

Not everyone accepted Pasteur's findings, but some pioneers did – notably a German doctor named **Robert Koch**. In 1876, he and his research team made an important breakthrough. They found the bacterium that was causing anthrax (a disease that affected animals and humans). This was the first time anyone had identified the specific **microbe** that causes a particular disease.

Over the next 20 years, Koch and other scientists identified more bacteria causing individual diseases and this led to the development of vaccines to prevent them.

This finally persuaded people that bad air was not the cause of disease. For the first time, doctors understood what really did cause diseases and this revolutionised medicine in different ways. The diagram on the opposite page sums this up.

> **Reflect**
>
> **What was the impact of the Germ Theory?**
>
> Read both pages and explain why the Germ Theory was a turning point in the history of medicine.

The significance of Pasteur and the Germ Theory

Before Pasteur

Miasma theory of disease

By 1800, the main explanation of disease was **bad air** or **miasma**. This old idea made even more sense in the mid-1800s when towns were more crowded and filthy than ever before and were also more disease ridden.

Spontaneous generation

In the nineteenth century, using microscopes, scientists could see that rubbish was covered with bacteria. They could see germs on everything! The popular theory was that decaying matter was **creating these bacteria**. This was the theory of spontaneous generation.

Pasteur's ideas

Pasteur's Germ Theory argued that:
- Bacteria were not created by decaying matter, the bacteria **caused** the decay. Pasteur therefore challenged the theory of spontaneous generation.
- Germs got into the decaying matter from the air as germs were literally all around us all the time.
- Germs could cause wine or milk to go bad. They also got into humans and caused disease.

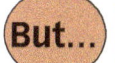

But... It was only a theory – it had to be proved and that took time.

And, though Pasteur made the breakthrough, others turned it into lifesaving treatments.

Short-term impact

- Robert Koch was the first to link an individual bacterium to an individual disease.
- Once specific bacteria had been linked to specific diseases, vaccines were developed to prevent them.
- Joseph Lister used carbolic spray to perform the first antiseptic surgery.

Long-term impact

New treatments: in the late 1800s, scientists developed the first chemical drugs (e.g. sulphonamides) and, in the 1930s, the first antibiotic (e.g. penicillin) that killed bacteria in the body was discovered.

Aseptic surgery: developed in the late nineteenth century. The aim was to make sure that operating theatres were germ free.

Improved public health: Pasteur's discovery encouraged councils and government to build sewers, to keep streets clean and to provide clean water.

Summarise

Draw your own version of this memory aid, then add your own examples to support each consequence.

Germ Theory made a **VAST** difference …

V = Vaccinations developed …, e.g. …

A = Acts to improve public health …, e.g. …

S = Surgery became safer …, e.g. …

T = Treatments improved …, e.g. …

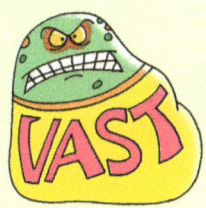

Topic 7: The development of the Germ Theory and its impact on the treatment of disease in Britain

7.2 Robert Koch and microbe hunting

Research & Record

What factors helped Robert Koch develop Pasteur's ideas?

The key factors that led to the development of the Germ Theory are summarised in the spider diagram below. Did the same factors help Koch in his hunt for microbes?

1. Complete this second spider diagram to show the factors that helped Koch develop Pasteur's ideas.
2. Study Source 1 on this page. Look very carefully at the cartoon. Can you spot two things that helped in Koch's hunt for microbes?

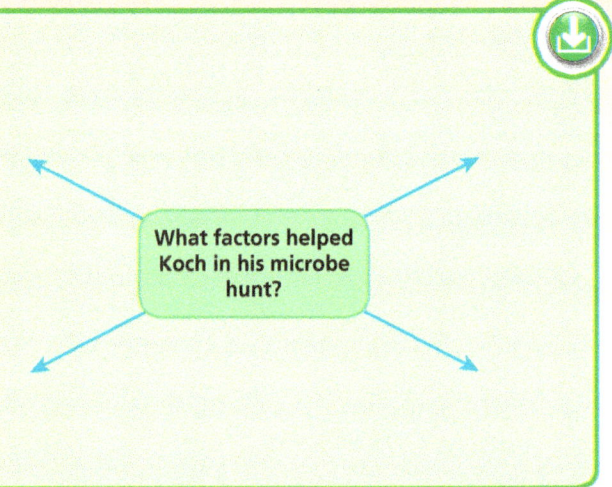

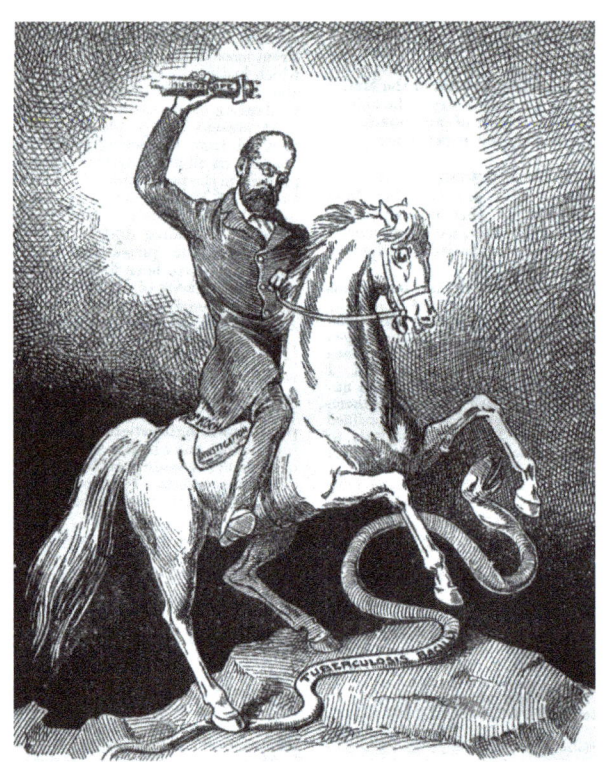

▶ **SOURCE 1** This cartoon from the 1880s shows Koch slaying the bacterium that causes tuberculosis (TB). TB spread rapidly in crowded conditions. It killed more people than any other disease in the nineteenth century. Germs were passed through the air by sneezing or coughing. The disease attacked the lungs and caused people to spit blood

How did Robert Koch play an important role in the battle against infectious diseases?

Robert Koch was a German doctor who became interested in Pasteur's work and began to study bacteria himself.

Rivals

Koch was just as ambitious as Pasteur and just as brilliant at detailed, painstaking work in his laboratory and working with a team of assistants. The two men saw each other as rivals, especially after the war between France and Germany in 1870–71, which was won by Germany. Both men wanted to be successful to glorify their country.

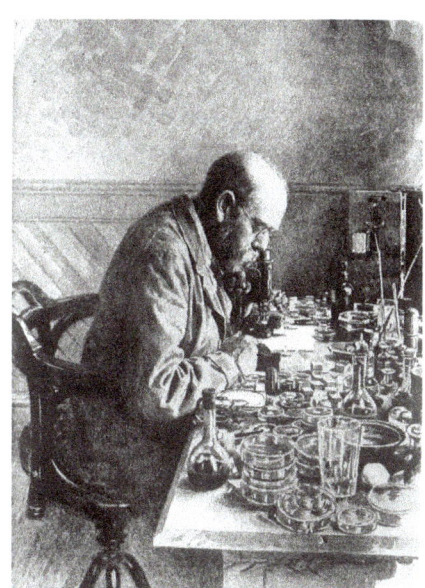

Breakthrough 1: Linking bacteria to specific diseases

Koch investigated anthrax, a disease affecting animals, and discovered the **specific bacterium** that causes the disease. This was the first time anyone had identified a specific germ that caused a particular disease. It was also the long-awaited final proof that Pasteur's Germ Theory was correct.

Breakthrough 2: Making it easier to study bacteria

Koch then developed a method of **staining bacteria** to make them easier to study. They could be photographed using a new, high-quality photographic lens.

Other scientists copied Koch's methods to discover bacteria that caused other diseases.

Breakthrough 3: Studying human disease

Pasteur used Koch's findings to develop a vaccine against anthrax (see page 54). Koch decided to get ahead again by becoming the first man to discover the specific germ that causes a human disease. He investigated the deadly disease of tuberculosis (TB, see Source 1). The TB bacterium was so small that it had been missed by other scientists so far, but Koch found a way of staining even such a tiny bacterium so that it stood out from other bacteria and human tissue.

This was the major breakthrough he had been searching for. His research team followed this up by discovering the specific bacterium that causes **cholera** (another feared disease).

Other scientists joined in the microbe hunt. By 1900, different teams had found the bacteria that caused other killer diseases, including typhoid, pneumonia, meningitis, plague and **dysentery**.

7.3 Vaccinations, magic bullets and everyday treatments

Research & Record

What impact did vaccinations and magic bullets have on ways of treating and preventing the spread of disease?

The development of the Germ Theory and the identification of bacteria that caused specific diseases led to improved ways of preventing and treating disease. However, people did not benefit immediately from all of these changes. Using the information on pages 54 and 55, record which areas of medicine progressed quickly and which areas were slower to change.

Area of medicine	Evidence that change happened quickly	Evidence that change occurred at a slower pace
Preventing disease		
Treating illness		

Pasteur discovers new vaccinations

Pasteur was determined to match Koch's discoveries and so built up a research team to make faster progress.

The chickens who did not die

The team started work trying to help the farming industry because an epidemic of chicken cholera was killing many thousands of chickens. In 1880, Pasteur left one of his team, Charles Chamberland, to inoculate a batch of chickens with the germ that caused chicken cholera, but Chamberland forgot and then the laboratory closed for the summer. When Chamberland came back, he finally inoculated the chickens, expecting them to die from cholera. They did not!

Pasteur solved the riddle of the chickens that didn't die! He realised that the germs left over the summer had weakened and were not strong enough to kill the chickens, but instead they protected the chickens from a strong dose of cholera. When people said it had been a lucky discovery, he replied 'No! Chance only favours prepared minds.'

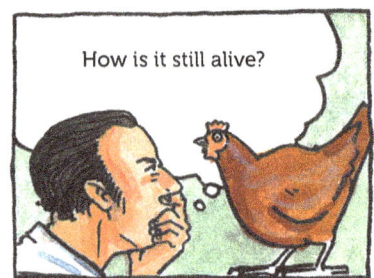

Anthrax vaccine

Now Pasteur could create other vaccines. At first, he continued to work on animals, producing a vaccine against anthrax. He tested this successfully in a public experiment and the news spread rapidly around Europe.

Rabies vaccine

After his success with vaccines against animal diseases, Pasteur turned to human diseases. He investigated rabies, testing his vaccine successfully on dogs, but did not know if it would work on people. The chance to find out came in 1885, when he tested his vaccine on Joseph Meister, a boy who had been bitten by a rabid dog. If the vaccine did not work, the boy would die. Pasteur gave Joseph thirteen injections over a two-week period. Joseph survived.

Other scientists follow

Now, other scientists set to work to follow Pasteur and find vaccines that could prevent other human diseases. Their successes included vaccines against: typhoid (1896), tuberculosis (1906), diphtheria (1913), tetanus (1927), measles (1950s) and polio (1950s).

Paul Ehrlich discovers the first chemical cures or 'magic bullets'

In 1909, **Paul Ehrlich** (who had been part of Koch's research team) developed the first chemical cure for a disease. This was Salvarsan 606, which he called a **'magic bullet'** because it homed in on and destroyed the harmful bacteria that caused syphilis. Before this, mercury had been used – it was dangerous and ineffective. Syphilis caused painful sores to develop, weakened bones (the nose could collapse) and could lead to heart disease and death. He did not know how it worked but, within three years, Salvarsan cured 10,000 people.

However, it wasn't until more than 20 years later, in the 1930s, that **Gerhard Domagk** developed the second chemical magic bullet, Prontosil, which could cure blood poisoning.

Scientists then discovered that the important chemical in these cures was sulphonamide and drug companies then developed more sulphonamide cures for diseases such as pneumonia.

But magic bullets could not kill the germs that caused most infections, so they were not a complete solution.

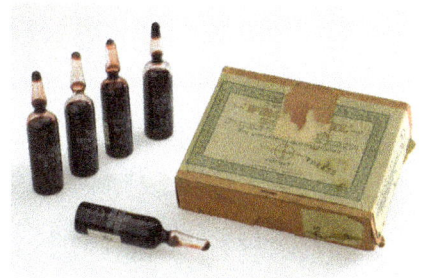

▲ **SOURCE 1** Prontosil, 'magic bullets'

Everyday medical treatments and remedies

Despite all this, most people were treated at home in traditional ways.

Home remedies

Everyday treatments were slow to develop. Until 1900, the improvements in medical knowledge did not lead immediately to effective new treatments. The most common form of treatment continued to be home remedies. In many ways, treatments used by most people had a lot in common with medieval remedies. The suggested cure for tuberculosis (before vaccines were introduced) was to breathe into a freshly dug hole in the turf or to inhale the breath of stallions and cows.

Patent medicines

If home remedies did not work, people bought 'patent' medicines, often known as 'cure-alls'. Patent medicines were big business, largely thanks to massive advertising campaigns by their manufacturers. Thomas Holloway became a multi-millionaire selling pills containing ginger, soap and aloes, a very powerful purgative, until a court case against him in the 1860s.

There was no control over the manufacturing standards or the ingredients in patent medicines until the 1880s, so false claims about their effectiveness were made without fear of prosecution. Addiction, deaths and illnesses resulting from overdoses were common. In the 1880s, governments introduced laws controlling the use of harmful ingredients, but the medicines still contained lard, wax and turpentine – and still claimed to cure all illnesses!

▼ **SOURCE 2** A nineteenth-century advertisement for Holloway's ointment. Different versions of the ointment were claimed to treat everything from gout, rheumatism, ulcers, tumours and scrofula to burns, sore breasts, ringworm and insect bites

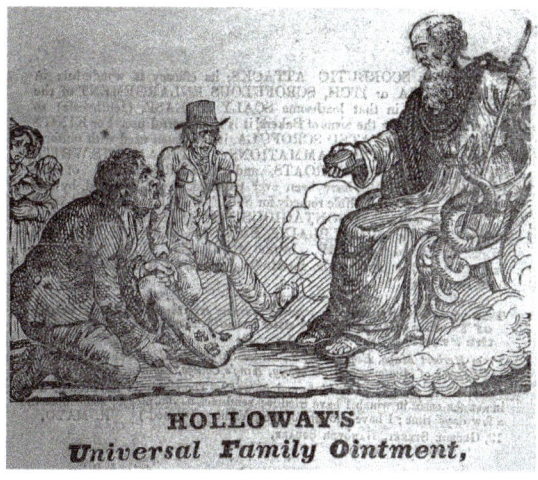

Topic 8: A revolution in surgery

8.1 The problems facing surgeons in the early 1800s

Research & Record

What were the main problems facing surgeons in the early 1800s?

1. Look at Source 1. Fill in a table like this. How is each problem shown in the source?
2. Read page 57. Why didn't these anaesthetics fully solve the problem of pain?

Problem	Clues that suggest this in the source
Surgeons were not respected. They were seen as butchers or torturers	The list of approved surgeons in the background contains names such as Samuel Sawbone and …
Painful for the patient due to lack of effective anaesthetics	
Infection could spread easily due to lack of effective antiseptics and a crowded, unclean operating environment	
Very basic technology, surgical tools and equipment	
High death rates (patients died from the shock of pain, blood loss and infection)	

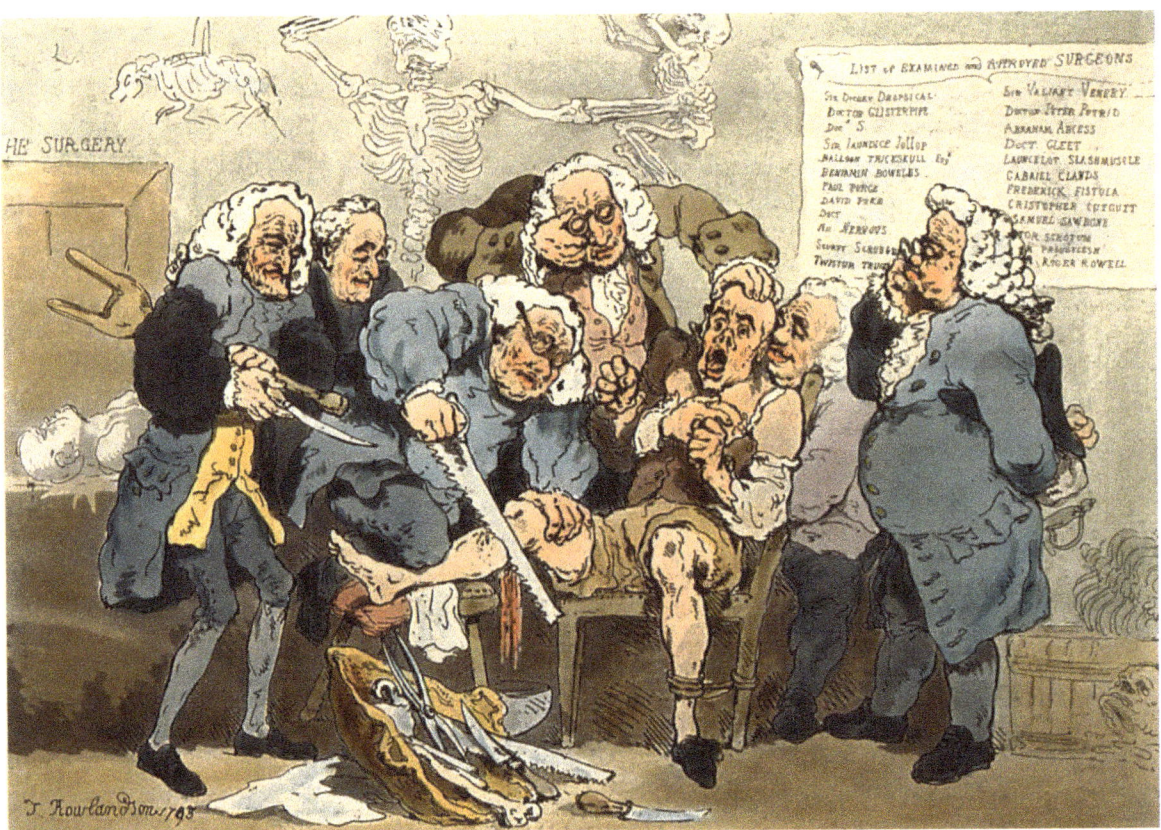

▲ **SOURCE 1** A cartoon showing an amputation, published in 1793

Early anaesthetics

Through the centuries, surgeons tried various ways to deal with pain.

- In the Middle Ages, they used herbs such as mandrake and hemlock. Both could kill if too much was used.
- In the Renaissance period, they tried alcohol and opium. However, alcohol did not make the patient totally unconscious and opium could kill through overdose.

Speed

However, nothing was totally effective, so the only way to reduce pain was speed. The patient was held or tied down by the surgeon's assistants while the surgeon operated as quickly as possible. At the Battle of Borodino in 1812, Napoleon's surgeon, Dubois, amputated 200 limbs in 24 hours. Surgeons prided themselves on their speed. Speed was one sign of a good surgeon.

The danger of speed!

Speed could also cause problems. Robert Liston, a famous London surgeon, once amputated a leg in two-and-a-half minutes but worked so fast that he accidentally cut off his patient's testicles as well.

During another high-speed operation, Liston amputated the fingers of his assistant and slashed the coat of a spectator who, fearing that he had been stabbed, dropped dead with fright. And both the assistant and the patient died of infection after the operation.

Improved anaesthetics

The late 1700s and 1800s saw an explosion of interest in chemistry. Scientists studied the properties of different chemicals. They also found out that some chemicals could have effects on the human body. This resulted in improved anaesthetics.

Laughing gas

In 1799, Sir Humphry Davy discovered that 'laughing gas' (properly called nitrous oxide) reduced the sensation of pain. He suggested that it might be useful in surgery or dentistry. However, it did not make patients completely unconscious. Also, when an American dentist, Horace Wells, used it in a public demonstration, his patient was in agony. This damaged confidence in laughing gas as an anaesthetic.

Ether

In 1846, ether was used as an anaesthetic in an operation in America to remove a neck tumour. A year later, in 1847, ether was used by Robert Liston in London to anaesthetise a patient during a leg amputation. Ether worked better than anything else so far. However, ether also had drawbacks.

- It was difficult to inhale.
- It irritated the eyes and lungs, causing coughing and sickness.
- It could catch fire if exposed to a flame.
- It had a vile smell that took ages to go away.
- It was stored in large, heavy bottles so was difficult to carry around.

Summarise

Surgeons in the Middle Ages and the Renaissance period faced a **PILE** of problems …

P = Pain
I = Infection
L = Loss of blood
E = Environment to operate in was unclean

8.1 The problems facing surgeons in the early 1800s

8.2 James Simpson and chloroform

Research & Record

What factors helped and hindered the use of chloroform?

1. Fill in a table like this to identify and explain which factors helped in the development of chloroform as an anaesthetic. You should be able to identify at least four factors that played a role. Make sure you include factors that helped overcome opposition to chloroform. Use pages 58 and 59 to help you.

2. There was opposition to the use of chloroform. Identify a reason from Source 3 and then try to identify and explain one other reason for opposition from page 59.

Factor	Explanation of how it helped
Science & technology	Interest in chemistry led scientists to study the effects of chemicals on the human body

The discovery of chloroform

James Simpson was Professor of Midwifery at Edinburgh University. He had used ether as a painkiller but was searching for a better anaesthetic. One evening in 1847, he and several colleagues sat around a table experimenting with different chemicals to see what anaesthetic effects they had. Simpson wrote later:

> ▼ **SOURCE 1**
>
> I poured some of the chloroform fluid into tumblers in front of my assistants, Dr Keith and Dr Duncan, and myself. Before sitting down to supper, we all inhaled the fluid, and were all 'under the table' in a minute or two, to my wife's consternation and alarm.

Simpson realised that he had discovered a very effective anaesthetic. **Chloroform** was faster-acting and gentler than ether. Within days, he started using it to help women in childbirth and in other operations. He wrote articles about his discovery and other surgeons started to use it in their operations.

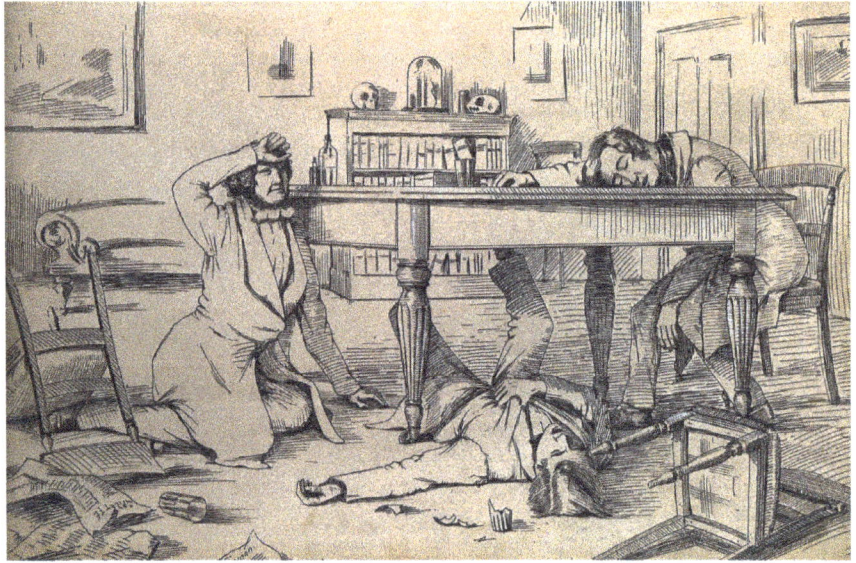

◄ **SOURCE 2** Simpson and friends recovering from the effects of chloroform. A drawing made in 1857. Simpson is on the left

Opposition to chloroform

There was a lot of opposition to chloroform for several different reasons.

Reason 1: Chloroform was new and untested

No one knew if there would be long-term side effects on the bodies or minds of patients. They also did not know what dose to give to different patients.

When Hannah Greener died during a routine operation (see Source 3) this scared surgeons and gave opponents of anaesthetics powerful evidence of the dangers of chloroform.

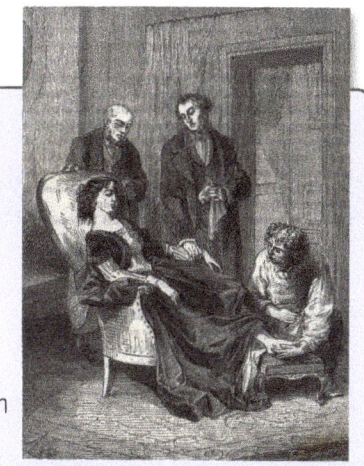

▶ **SOURCE 3** This engraving shows the death of Hannah Greener in 1848. She died from an overdose of chloroform while she was having a toenail removed

Reason 2: 'Pain is good'

Some people were opposed to the use of anaesthetics to ease pain on principle.

▼ **SOURCE 4A** Letter to the medical journal *The Lancet* in 1853:

It is a most unnatural practice. The pain and sorrow of labour exert a most powerful and useful influence upon the religious and moral character of women and upon all their future relations in life.

▼ **SOURCE 4B** Letter to the medical journal *The Lancet* in 1849:

The infliction [of pain] has been invented by the Almighty God. Pain may even be considered a blessing of the Gospel, and being blessed admits to being made either well or ill.

▼ **SOURCE 4C** A quotation from Army Chief of Medical Staff, 1854:

… the smart use of the knife is a powerful stimulant and it is much better to hear a man bawl lustily than to see him sink silently into the grave.

Reason 3: It increased the risk of infection

Anaesthetics did not make surgery safer. With a patient asleep, doctors soon attempted more complex operations. They therefore carried infections deeper into the body and caused more loss of blood. The number of people dying from surgery increased from the 1850s to the early 1870s, which is known as surgery's 'Black Period'. In the 1870s, some surgeons stopped using chloroform because they were concerned about the high death rate (1 in 2500 operations). They returned to using ether mixed with nitrous oxide.

How was opposition overcome?

James Simpson played a leading role in promoting chloroform. He used it regularly and carefully communicated to other doctors how it could be used safely.

Then, a breakthrough came when Queen Victoria was given chloroform during the delivery of her eighth child in 1853. She publicly praised 'that blessed chloroform'. With the support of the Queen, opposition to anaesthetics was doomed!

Consequences of chloroform

In the short term, developments in anaesthetics allowed more complex operations. Surgeons could work more slowly and carefully without fear that their patients might die from shock. However, this also increased the risk of infection (described in Reason 3), so it was not a totally positive outcome.

In the longer term, the power of chloroform encouraged others to search for even better anaesthetics.

- Other chemicals were used which relaxed muscles as well as simply putting patients to sleep.
- Local anaesthetics were developed which numbed pain in one specific area of the body.

This took time, but Simpson's use of chloroform had been the turning point.

8.3 Antiseptics: Lister and carbolic acid

Research & Record

How did Joseph Lister change surgery?
Use pages 60 and 61 to fill in a bingo card like the one below. It should help you collect evidence to:

a prove the significance of Lister's work
b identify the factors that helped Lister
c explain why Lister also faced opposition.

Lister Bingo		
What new development had made surgery even more dangerous by 1860?	**By what percentage** did deaths from amputations fall when Lister used carbolic acid?	**How** was carbolic acid used before Lister used it as an antiseptic?
Give 2 examples of liquids used to keep wounds clean before Lister	**Which 2 famous scientists** helped Lister's ideas become more widely accepted?	**Give 2 reasons** why Lister was partly to blame for the opposition he faced
List 3 dangerous things that surgeons did before Lister changed surgery	**List 3 examples** of how Lister improved his methods	**List 3 reasons** people opposed Lister's methods

What was surgery like before Lister?

An operation without anaesthetics was horrible. Patients sometimes died just from the shock of the pain. However, many more patients died from something much less dramatic – infection after the operation.

Doctors knew infection could be fatal. They had used liquids such as wine and vinegar to keep wounds clean for centuries. Paré had developed his own treatment (see page 37).

However, before Pasteur's Germ Theory, no one knew what was causing the infection, so surgeons did things that seem obviously dangerous to us today.

- They reused bandages, spreading gangrene and skin infections from patient to patient.
- They did not wash their hands before an operation.
- They did not **sterilise** their equipment.
- Some surgeons operated wearing old blood- and pus-stained clothes.

This was how they had done operations for years. It was what they were used to.

What inspired Lister to look for new ways to stop infection?

Joseph Lister was one of the outstanding surgeons of the nineteenth century. He was keenly interested in science and applying it to medicine. He had researched gangrene – trying to understand the way that infection spread.

Most importantly, he knew all about Pasteur's work on the Germ Theory. It was Pasteur's work that drove Lister to look for ways to kill bacteria in the wound.

His solution was carbolic acid.

Where did Lister's idea of using carbolic acid come from?

The answer is sewage! In 1864, Lister observed how carbolic acid was used to reduce the smell of sewage that was used to fertilise the land. He noted how it also destroyed the parasites that usually infect cattle feeding on such land.

Lister experimented with carbolic acid to treat people with compound fractures (where the bone breaks through the skin). Infection often developed in these open wounds. Lister applied carbolic acid to the wound and used bandages soaked in it. He found that the wounds healed and did not develop gangrene.

What impact did Lister's work have in the short term?

Lister went on to use carbolic acid when he performed amputations. It dramatically reduced deaths from infection (see Source 1). In 1867, Lister published his results, showing the value of using carbolic acid. He also worked at improving his method so that bacteria were being killed at every stage of an operation.

▼ SOURCE 1 From Lister's record of amputations

	Total amputations	Died	Percentage who died
1864–66 (without antiseptics)	35	16	45.7%
1867–70 (with antiseptics)	40	6	15.0%

Handwashing with carbolic before operations to avoid the surgeon carrying infection into wounds.

A **carbolic spray** to kill germs in the air around the operating table.
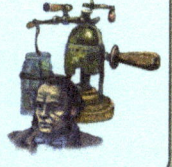

Antiseptic ligatures to tie up blood vessels after surgery.
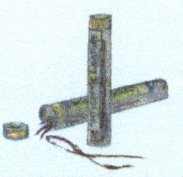

Why was there opposition to antiseptics?

It was unpleasant
Carbolic spray soaked the operating theatre. It cracked the surgeon's skin and made everything smell unpleasant.

Pasteur's ideas spread slowly
Even some trained surgeons found it hard to accept that tiny organisms were all around, causing disease. One surgeon joked with his assistants to shut the door of the operating room 'in case one of Mr Lister's microbes flew in'.

It slowed down operations
The new precautions caused extra work. Despite anaesthetics, surgeons still thought speed was essential – often because of the problem of bleeding.

Lister was not a showman
Unlike Pasteur, Lister did not give impressive public displays. In fact, he appeared cold and arrogant, and he criticised other surgeons. Many surgeons regarded him as a fanatic.

It did not always work
Some surgeons tried Lister's methods but did not achieve the same results. This was usually because they were less careful, but that did not stop them criticising Lister.

Lister changed his techniques
He did this because he wanted to find a substance that would work as well as carbolic spray, but without the corrosion that it caused. His critics simply said he was changing his methods because they did not work.

How was opposition overcome?

By Lister's determination
Lister's demonstrations and teachings helped to overcome opposition. In 1869, he became Professor of Clinical Surgery at Edinburgh University. Over the next eight years, he demonstrated his methods to over 1500 medical students. In 1877, he moved to King's College Hospital, London to train young surgeons.

With help from others
Then came a link to another great name in medical history. In 1878, Robert Koch discovered the bacterium which caused septicaemia (blood poisoning). This gave a great boost to Lister's ideas. By the end of the century, they were widely accepted.

Once the opposition was overcome, Lister's methods marked a turning point in surgery.

8.4 Aseptic surgery and better surgical procedures

Research & Record

What was the long-term significance of Lister's work?

Read page 62. Find the following:
- **One example** of another individual who helped surgery improve.
- **Two examples** of more ambitious surgery which resulted from Lister's work.
- **Three examples** of measures introduced to reduce the risk of infection (aseptic surgery).

'A true glove story'

Caroline Hampton was an operating-theatre nurse. She developed a skin problem from the chemicals used to disinfect hands before operations. She showed her hands to William Halsted, the surgeon, and he arranged for the Goodyear Rubber Company (famous for car tyres!) to make a pair of thin rubber gloves to protect Caroline's hands. Within a year, the nurse and the surgeon were married! And Halsted spread the idea of wearing rubber gloves during operations.

Antiseptic surgery leads to aseptic surgery

Lister's methods which killed germs on the wound was called antiseptic surgery. By the late 1890s, this had developed into **aseptic surgery**, which meant removing all possible germs from the operating theatre. To ensure absolute cleanliness:

- Operating theatres and hospitals were carefully cleaned.
- All instruments were steam-sterilised.
- Surgeons no longer wore ordinary clothes but surgical gowns and face masks.
- Sterilised rubber gloves were introduced (see panel).

Surgery becomes more ambitious

With two of the basic problems of surgery now solved, surgeons attempted more ambitious operations.

- The first successful operation to remove an infected appendix came in the 1880s. Surgery on the small intestine, to stop the spread of cancer, also started around this time.
- The first heart operation was carried out in 1896, when surgeons repaired a heart damaged by a stab wound.

James Simpson and Joseph Lister had made major contributions. Their work helped make such operations possible. As surgeons started to perform more complex and safer operations, their status improved.

Summarise

1. Can you remember the four problems that surgeons faced in the early 1800s? What did PILE stand for? (Go back to page 56 if you can't remember.)
2. Explain how three of these problems had been tackled by 1900. Use this AAA memory aid to help you.

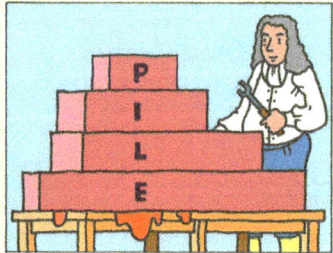
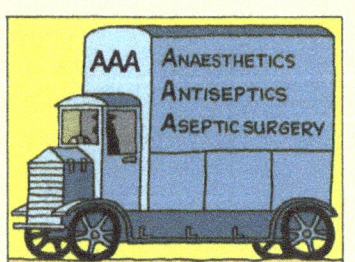

Apply ▶ Exam Practice

Revisiting Question 1

Study Source 1. How useful is Source 1 for a historian studying surgery in the late nineteenth century? **(8 marks)**

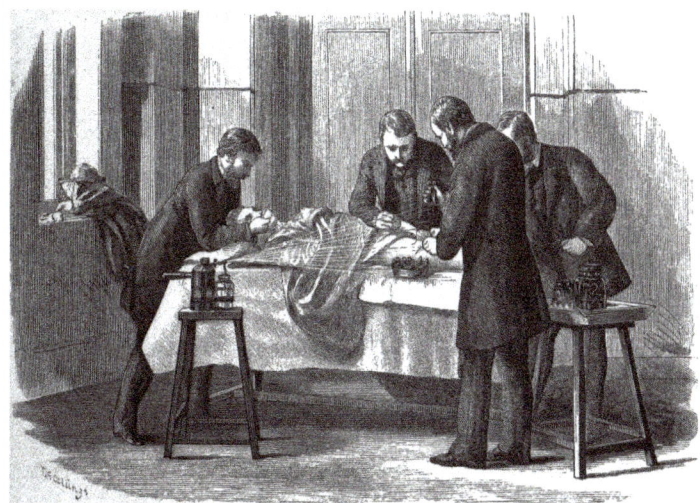

▲ **SOURCE 1** This picture shows an operation taking place while a carbolic spray disinfects the area. One assistant is using chloroform to anaesthetise the patient, another is mopping up blood with a sponge. The picture comes from a textbook for surgeons called *Antiseptic Surgery*, produced by William Watson Cheyne in 1882. Cheyne was an experienced surgeon at King's College Hospital, London (where Lister worked from 1877) and was a keen supporter of Lister's methods

Exam Tip

Take responsibility

Remind yourself of the CPK advice on page 33 about how to approach this type of question.

C Look carefully at the **content** of the source. Explain how the source shows the use of anaesthetics and antiseptics.

P Use the **provenance** of the source. Explain why the author is a useful source of information – note that he was an experienced surgeon who worked at King's College Hospital and would have been very knowledgeable about Lister's methods. Explain the significance of the date (1882) and link this to your contextual knowledge – by this date carbolic spray was being widely used, but aseptic techniques were still being developed.

K Use your **contextual knowledge**. This source shows that aseptic surgery had not yet been fully developed. Some attempt is being made to keep the operating environment clean, as we can see one assistant mopping up blood with a sponge, but other aseptic techniques have yet to be introduced. Can you remember aseptic techniques that were introduced later to reduce the risk of infection? If you can't, look back at page 62 before you plan your answer.

Apply ▶ Exam Practice

Revisiting Question 2

Explain the significance of the work of Joseph Lister in the development of surgery. **(8 marks)**

Exam Tip

Take responsibility

Use your bingo card from page 60 and the notes you have just made. Also remind yourself of the advice on page 35 about how to approach this type of question.

Aim for two developed paragraphs:

Paragraph 1: explain how Lister changed surgery in the short term.

Paragraph 2: explain the longer-term significance of Lister's work.

Topic 9: Improvements in public health

9.1 Public health problems in industrial Britain

Research & Record

Why was public health so poor in industrial Britain?

1. Use the case studies on pages 64 and 65 to record public health problems. You should come up with a long list. Aim to identify at least ten problems.
2. Identify three similarities between the cholera epidemics of the nineteenth century and the Great Plague of London in 1665.

Case Study 1: The Great Stink of 1858

By the 1850s, over 2.5 million people lived in London. It was the largest and wealthiest city in the world, but it was also very unhealthy.

Many Londoners got their drinking water from the River Thames, even though the river was also where they dumped their rubbish – including dead animals and chemicals from factories based by the river. There was no sewage system so human waste ended up in the river as well.

The summer of 1858 was very hot. A thick layer of sewage lay on the water. As temperatures topped 30°C, the smell of the river became unbearable. It became known as the 'Great Stink'. In the Houses of Parliament, MPs found it impossible to use the rooms overlooking the river.

At that time, many people still believed that bad air (miasma) caused disease, so they treated the curtains with chloride of lime. It had little impact and the awful smell remained.

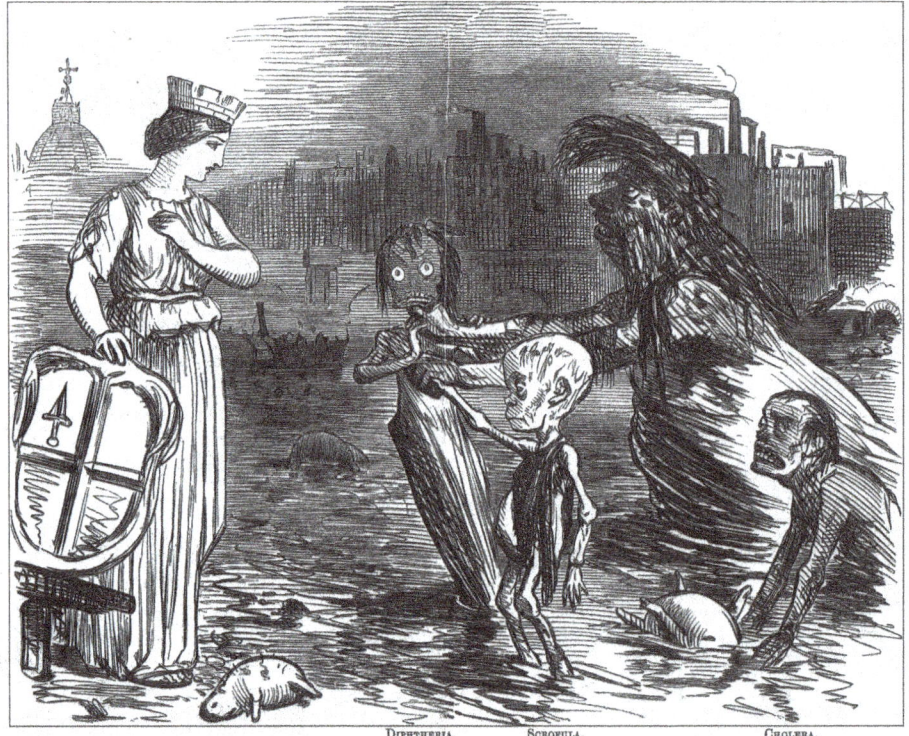

▼ **SOURCE 1** This cartoon was published in *Punch* magazine in June 1858, during the Great Stink. The River Thames is shown as a filthy old man with diseased and deformed offspring

Case Study 2: Cholera epidemics

One result of these awful conditions was more frequent outbreaks of cholera. There were four major epidemics between 1831 and 1865. Cholera was as frightening as plague had been in previous centuries. It was caused by drinking unclean water. Violent sickness and diarrhoea led to severe dehydration and death. It could kill people in less than a day. The epidemic of 1848–49 killed 53,293 people. Cholera spread because germs from cesspits infected the water supply. But people did not know this. So responses to cholera were a familiar mix of old and new, common sense and **supernatural** remedies (see panel).

Methods used to prevent the spread of cholera in the 1830s and 1840s

- To protect against bad air: burning barrels of tar; inhaling vinegar; smoking cigars
- Praying to God or wearing lucky charms
- Taking patent medicines that 'guaranteed' protection
- Burning the clothes and bedding of those who had the disease
- Quarantine – guards stopped people living in poverty from entering the city

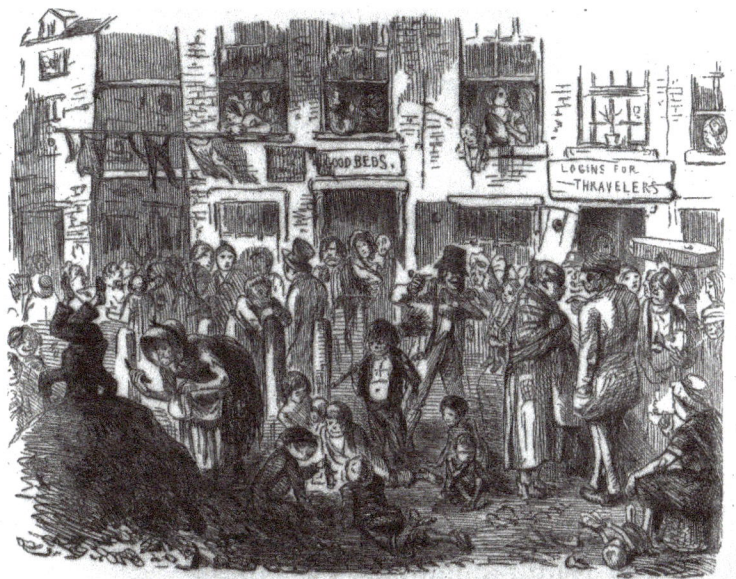
A COURT FOR KING CHOLERA.

◀ **SOURCE 2** A cartoon published in 1852 in *Punch* magazine. A court was an enclosed area of housing, often dark and over-populated

Case Study 3: Life expectancy in cities

In 1842, Edwin Chadwick published an important report on poverty. (You will read more about his work on page 66). His report showed the average age at death among different groups of people in 1840. Liverpool was chosen as an example of a large, rapidly growing industrial town. Rutland was chosen as a country area. The results were truly shocking. Working-class people in Liverpool lived, on average, to age 15! In Rutland, the average life expectancy of a working-class person was 38 years. It is not hard to explain these differences.

- **Living conditions** in industrial cities were worse than in the Middle Ages. Badly ventilated houses were crammed close together. Families shared privies (outside toilets). Diseases like cholera spread quickly.
- **Working conditions** were also harmful. Twelve-hour working days were common in hot and dirty workshops, surrounded by dangerous machinery.
- **Fresh food** was hard to get or expensive because it had to be brought in to town by horse and cart.
- **Doctors** charged fees, so less affluent people could not afford to see one.
- **Water supply** was the most fundamental problem of all. It was hard to get fresh, clean drinking water.

▼ **SOURCE 3**

Gentry or professionals

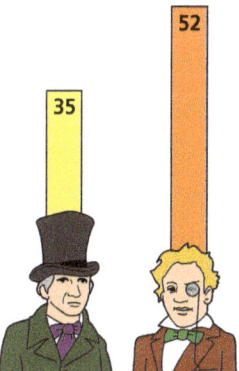
Liverpool 35 Rutland 52

Labourers or artisans

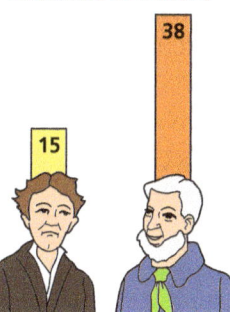
Liverpool 15 Rutland 38

9.2 The factors behind public health improvement: Part 1

Research & Record

What factors played a role in early public health improvements?

Use a table like this to explain how individuals, chance events and government played a role in improving public health.

NB: You will add to your table after reading pages 66 and 67, so leave lots of space. You will also find out about science and technology on the next page too. Finally, leave column 3 (your evaluation) until you have completed all factors.

Factor	Explanation: How did it influence improvements?	Evaluation: How important was this factor?
Individuals	Chadwick ... Snow ...	
Chance	The cholera epidemics ...	
Government (local and national)	The 1848 Public Health Act ...	
Science & technology		

The work of Edwin Chadwick

The shocking conditions in Britain's industrial cities led a civil servant, Edwin Chadwick, to compile his 'Report on the Sanitary Conditions of the Labouring Population' in 1842.

He found that:
1. Those living in poverty lived in dirty, overcrowded conditions.
2. This caused a huge amount of illness.
3. Many people were too sick to work and so became poorer still.
4. Therefore, other people had to pay higher taxes to help people living in poverty.

His solution was for the government to reform public health. He said that the government could cut taxes and save money in the long run by:
1. improving drainage and sewers
2. removing refuse from streets and houses
3. providing clean water supplies
4. appointing medical officers in each area to check these reforms were implemneted.

The impact of cholera

There was much opposition to Chadwick's report. Many local tax-payers did not want to pay for improvements and local councils did not want the national government interfering in local matters. However, as cholera spread across Europe in 1847, fear grew in Britain of many thousands of deaths to come. Therefore, the government finally followed Chadwick's recommendations and passed the Public Health Act in the hope this would reduce the impact of cholera.

The 1848 Public Health Act

The major points in this reform were:

- The National Board of Health was set up.
- In towns where the death rate was very high, the government could force the local council to make public health improvements to water supply and **sewerage**, and appoint a Medical Officer of Health.
- Local councils were encouraged to make public health improvements. They could collect taxes (called rates) to pay for this, provided they had the support of local rate-payers.

However, the 1848 Act was not compulsory. It encouraged change, but it did not force councils to make changes. Only 103 towns set up local boards of health. The majority of local councils did little to improve public health. To make matters worse, the National Board of Health, set up to oversee reforms, was abolished in 1854 after only six years.

The work of John Snow

John Snow was another important individual in the story of public health improvements. In 1849, he published a book putting forward his view that cholera spread through water, not in 'bad air'. His suggestion was mocked by many doctors.

The research

In 1854, another cholera outbreak gave him the chance to prove his theory right. Cholera had killed over 500 people around Broad Street in central London, near to Snow's surgery, in just ten days.

This led Snow to map out the deaths in detail. He linked all the deaths to a single water pump on Broad Street.

He found that a workhouse prison near Broad Street had virtually no cases of cholera because it had its own well. In contrast, Snow discovered that a lady from another part of London had died from cholera because she enjoyed the Broad Street water so much that she had it delivered to her home.

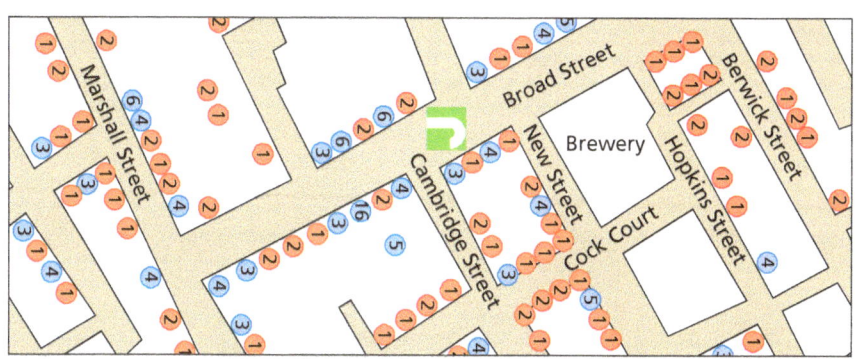

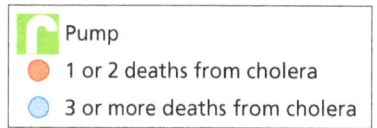

◀ **SOURCE 1** A copy of part of Snow's map detailing deaths in the Broad Street area

The solution

Snow wrote a report on his findings. His evidence was so strong that the handle of the Broad Street water pump was taken away to stop people getting water from it. There were no more deaths. It was later discovered that a **cesspool**, only a metre away from the pump, was leaking into the drinking water. A woman living in Broad Street whose baby had contracted cholera had dumped a nappy into the cesspool, just three feet from the Broad Street water pump.

The impact

Snow had proved that clean water was essential for preventing the spread of cholera, but even this did not convince the government to act.

Many scientists still clung to the 'bad air' theory. Snow proved the link between the water and cholera, but could not explain *why* there was this link. It was not until after Pasteur published his Germ Theory that anyone could begin to understand exactly why the water was causing cholera.

There was a further cholera epidemic in 1865, which killed 14,000 people. But even this did not force the government to act. There were three main reasons why a new law was not passed.

- Wealthy people did not want to pay taxes to cover the cost of clean water supplies and sewers, which would benefit other people in the less affluent parts of their towns.
- Local councils did not want the national government interfering in how they ran their own towns.
- There was a strong belief in *laissez-faire* (governments should not interfere in people's lives) and self-help (that people should help themselves to live better lives). Governments were still not expected to play a major part in improving the living and working conditions of the people.

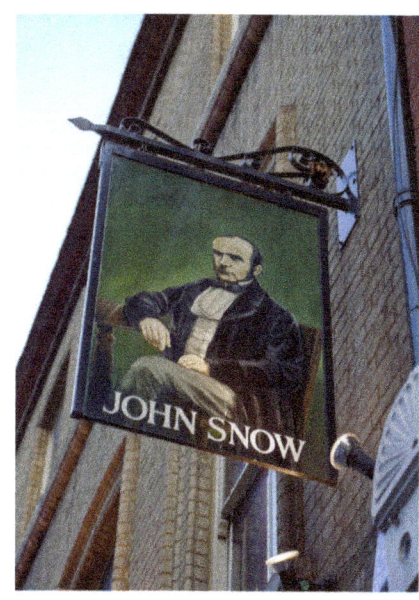

▼ This pub near the Broad Street pump named itself in honour of John Snow

9.3 The factors behind public health improvement: Part 2

Research & Record

What factors played the most important role in public health improvements?

Use the timeline below to complete column 3 of the table you started on page 66.

Think carefully about the words you use to evaluate the importance of each factor. Which factors were essential to public health improvement? Which factor was important?

Essential	No change could have happened without it
Important	Without it change might have been less widespread or significant
Minimal	Had only a little impact
No importance	No influence at all

1842 Chadwick's report
(see page 66) highlights the link between illness and poor living conditions.

1854 John Snow links cholera to infected water
(see page 67). His work showed the importance of using data to study epidemics. It also added to the pressure for clean water and effective sewerage systems.

1848 First Public Health Act
(see page 66) allows, but does not force, councils to make improvements.

1858 'The Great Stink'
(see page 64) added to the evidence that London needed a sewer system.

Summarise

The **SEWAGE** memory aid summarises Public Health changes in the nineteenth century.

- S = **S**ewers open
- E = **E**pidemics, e.g. cholera
- W = **W**ater unclean
- A = **A**cts by government, e.g. 1848 and 1875
- G = **G**erm Theory and Great Stink trigger action
- E = **E**ngineers improve sanitation, e.g. Bazalgette

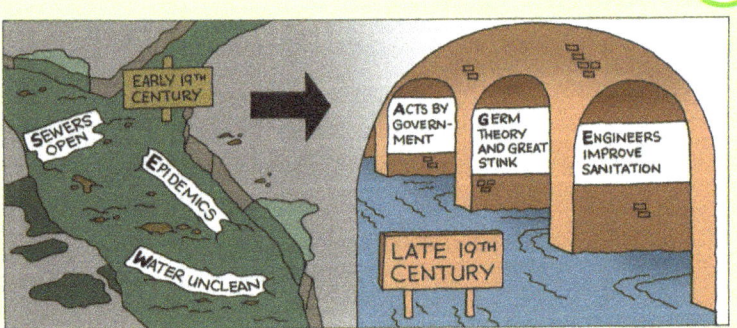

1860s Joseph Bazalgette organises the building of London's sewer system

In the 1850s, many people still believed that bad air (miasma) carried disease, so Londoners were scared by the Great Stink. This chance event forced MPs to take action to clean up the River Thames. They approved money to pay for a new sewage system for London.

It was a major engineering achievement which is still in use today. All London's sewage was pumped out of the city through:

- 83 miles of large sewers, built underground from brick
- 1100 miles of smaller connecting sewers from each street
- pumping stations at regular points to pump the sewage along the pipes.

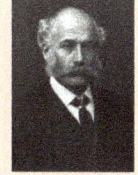

This project was led by **Joseph Bazalgette**. During the Industrial Revolution, there had been great improvements in technology and engineering. Bazalgette used what he had learned in railway building to design and manage this project.

Most of the work was complete by 1865 and it led to significant improvements in the public health of London. But there was no public health act to enforce improvements throughout the country.

1875 A new and more effective Public Health Act

The 1875 Public Health Act finally **forced** local councils to improve public health. After this turning point, it was compulsory for local councils in each city or town to:

- improve sewers and drainage
- provide fresh water supplies
- appoint medical officers and sanitary inspectors to inspect public health facilities.

1875 Octavia Hill shows how to provide healthy homes for working people

Octavia Hill started teaching children living in poverty when she was only fourteen. She was appalled by their homes. She bought three London slum houses in 1865 and cleaned them up to show others how to provide healthy homes for working people and stop overcrowding. Over time, she bought and improved over 2000 houses. This led to similar schemes elsewhere and she went on to campaign for laws which would force local councils to improve housing.

The Artisans' Dwellings Act

Octavia Hill's influence helped persuade the government to pass the 1875 Artisans' Dwelling Act, giving councils the power to knock down slum housing if it was believed to be unhealthy.

1860s Pasteur's Germ Theory

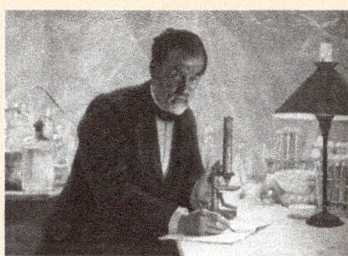

Pasteur proved that there was a link between dirt and disease. The theory that illness was caused by 'bad air' finally faded away. This was a turning point. Faced with scientific proof, people were more willing to pay taxes to cover the costs of cleaning up their towns and cities, and more councils accepted responsibility to improve public health.

1867 Working men get the vote

The number of voters doubled. Now, if politicians wanted to win elections, they had to promise to do things to help working men, not just the wealthy and middle classes. The 1870s and 1880s saw many new laws passed designed to improve the lives of ordinary people.

1875–1900 More laws to improve public health

Laws were passed to:

- stop the pollution of rivers (from which people got water)
- shorten working hours in factories for women and children
- make it illegal to put unhealthy additives in food
- make education compulsory.

9.4 Nineteenth century period review

Review

What factors led to improvements in medicine and public health during the nineteenth century?

Fill in a table like the one below to review the period. Use the cards at the bottom of the page to guide you.

Theme	Improvements during the nineteenth century	Key individuals	Other factors
Knowledge about the causes of illness	Reached a turning point. • From 1860s, the Germ Theory replaced bad air as an explanation for disease. • Microbes that cause individual diseases were identified.		
Treatments	More continuity than change. • Everyday treatments remained the same. Patent medicines often worthless. (NB: Chemical cures (magic bullets) and antibiotics did not appear until the twentieth century.)		
Methods of preventing disease	Significant improvements after 1860s. • Smallpox vaccination made compulsory. • Other vaccinations developed (e.g. anthrax, rabies).		
Surgery	Revolutionised after c1840. • Dealing with pain: anaesthetics (e.g. ether, chloroform). • Dealing with infection: use of carbolic acid; start of aseptic surgery.		
Public health	Improvements from c1840s. Major turning point in 1875. • 1860s London sewer system. • 1875 Public Health Act. Government forces councils to take responsibility.		

Factor: individuals
- Louis Pasteur
- Robert Koch
- James Simpson
- Joseph Lister
- John Snow
- Joseph Bazalgette

Factor: government
- Political change (vote given to working-class men)
- Public Health Act of 1848
- Public Health Act of 1875

Factor: chance
- Cholera epidemics
- The Great Stink

Factor: science & technology
- Better microscopes
- Improvements in chemistry
- Improvements in engineering

Factor: communication
- Jenner's work (read and used by …)
- Pasteur's work (read and used by …)

Apply ▶ Exam Practice

Revisiting questions 1–3

Question 1: How useful?

How useful is Source 1 to a historian studying public health in the nineteenth century? (8 marks)

▼ **SOURCE 1** This cartoon is called 'Death's Dispensary'. It was published in 1866

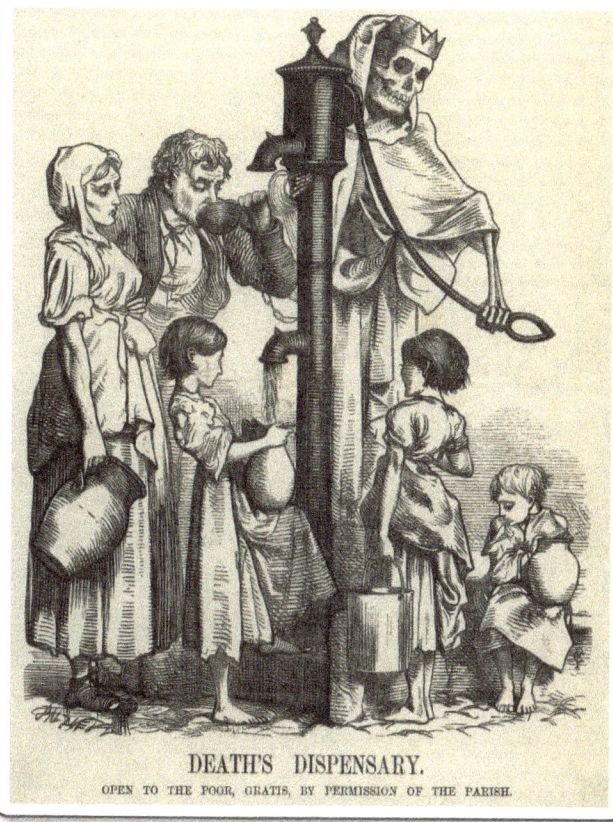

DEATH'S DISPENSARY.
OPEN TO THE POOR, GRATIS, BY PERMISSION OF THE PARISH.

Question 2: Significance

Explain the significance of the Germ Theory in the development of medicine in Britain. (8 marks)

Question 3: Comparisons

Explain two ways in which surgery at the time of Paré and surgery in the early 1800s were similar. Explain your answer with reference to both time periods. (8 marks)

Exam Tips

Question 1

Look again at the advice on how to approach this type of question on page 33.

Remember to focus on **why** the source is useful and to use your knowledge of the period.

- The date the cartoon was published is very important.
- It shows that by the 1860s people had accepted John Snow's theory that dirty water caused death.

It also shows that despite Snow's work, major public health improvements had still not been made. Remember that there were still cholera epidemics in the 1860s.

Question 2

Look again at the advice on how to approach this type of question on page 35.

Think about how Pasteur's work influenced a range of different areas of medicine.

Remember to explain the:

- Immediate impact – How did Pasteur's work change ideas about the cause of disease?
- Medium-term impact – How did the Germ Theory lead to microbe hunting, vaccinations and improvements in surgery?
- Longer-term significance – Why was Pasteur's research essential for the development of chemical cures and antibiotics?

Question 3

Look again at the advice on how to approach this type of question on page 43.

For a strong answer, do not write one paragraph describing surgery at the time of Paré and one paragraph about surgery at the end of the 1800s. Instead, make direct comparisons. For example:

- One paragraph could focus on the problem of pain.
- The second paragraph could focus on the problem of infection.

Period introduction: The twentieth century

10.1 Introducing ... Alexander Fleming – and the discovery of penicillin

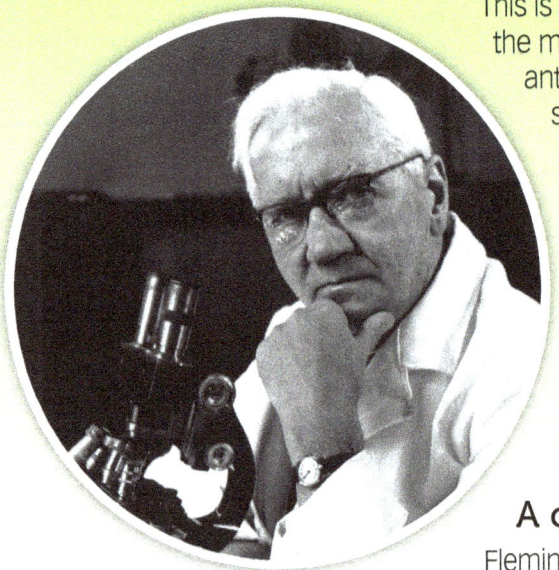

This is **Alexander Fleming**. He played a significant role in one of the most important medical breakthroughs – the first antibiotic. An antibiotic is a drug made from bacteria that kills other bacteria and so cures an infection or illness.

War wounds

During the First World War, Fleming was sent to France to study soldiers' wounds. He found that wounds infected with bacteria were not healed by chemical antiseptics. Many soldiers were dying from their infected wounds.

Back home, Fleming worked on finding a way to deal with these bacteria. Ten years later, in 1928, Fleming found what he had been seeking.

A chance discovery

Fleming was working at St Mary's Hospital, London. When he went on holiday, he left a pile of petri dishes containing bacteria on his laboratory bench. On his return, he sorted out the dishes and noticed mould on one of them. Around the mould, the bacteria had disappeared.

He looked closer through his microscope and could see that the areas where the bacteria had died were covered with a mould called penicillin. He did not know where it had come from – it must have blown in through the laboratory windows that were open while he was on holiday.

Fleming then carried out experiments with the penicillin mould.

- He discovered that if it was diluted, it killed bacteria without harming living cells.
- He made a list of the germs it killed.
- He used penicillin successfully to treat another scientist's eye infection.

However, it did not seem to work on deeper infections and it was taking ages to create enough penicillin to use in his experiments, so he stopped his research.

Communicating his findings

However, he did write up his experiments. In 1929, he published his research in a medical journal, but nobody thought his article was important. Fleming discussed penicillin's potential as an antiseptic, but he made no great claims for its role as a general antibiotic. Fleming had not used penicillin to heal major illnesses, nor done systematic tests on animals. It went largely unnoticed ... for now!

The opposite page summarises what happened next.

Reflect

How important was the work of Alexander Fleming?

Using these two pages:

1. Explain why Alexander Fleming's work was so important in the treatment of disease. Why was it a turning point? Think about how disease had been treated up until the 1920s.
2. Fleming may have discovered the properties of penicillin, but it needed other factors to turn his discovery into a life-saving drug. How many other factors can you identify? Make a list – you will need it for the task on page 74.

How has the treatment of disease developed since 1860?

Louis Pasteur

Pasteur publishes his Germ Theory in 1861. Doctors and scientists could now see the link between germs (microbes) and disease.

Robert Koch

Koch and his research team identify the specific microbes that were causing individual diseases. His methods also help others to do their own microbe hunting.

Joseph Lister

In 1872, Lister notices that the mould of bacteria called penicillin killed other bacteria. Years later, in 1884, he uses this mould to treat a nurse who had an infected wound. But Lister did not use it again. A miracle cure lay waiting for someone else to rediscover it.

Vaccinations

Scientists use Pasteur and Koch's work to develop a range of vaccinations.

Chemical cures

Scientists find magic bullets (chemicals) that kill particular infections inside the body.

In 1909, Paul Ehrlich developed Salvarsan 606, which destroys the bacteria that cause syphilis.

In the 1930s, Gerhard Domagk developed Prontisil, which kills the bacteria causing blood poisoning.

Sulphonamide drugs

The chemical in both Salvarsan 606 and Prontisil is **sulphonamide**.

Drug companies start to mass produce sulphonamide-based cures for diseases such as pneumonia and scarlet fever.

However, these magic bullets could not kill **staphylococcus** germs, which caused major infections and often killed people.

Alexander Fleming

Key ideas or discoveries

In 1928, Alexander Fleming discovers that penicillin kills bacteria.

He publishes his findings in 1929 but his ideas are not taken up straight away by other scientists.

Short-term impact

The development of penicillin – the first effective antibiotic.

In the 1930s, Howard Florey and Ernst Chain develop Fleming's idea into a medical treatment.

Penicillin becomes the first antibiotic.

Penicillin is used in the Second World War to treat Allied soldiers.

Long-term impact – Antibiotics for all

Penicillin and other antibiotics are mass produced by the **pharmaceutical industry**.

In Britain, after the Second World War, the government provides antibiotics free to anyone who needs them through the National Health Service.

The impact of antibiotics in modern medicine has been far reaching. It is no exaggeration to say that they have saved millions of lives.

Topic 10: Modern treatment of disease

10.2 The development of penicillin

Research & Record

How did factors affect the development of penicillin?

1. On page 72, you listed factors that were important in the development of penicillin. Use that list and these two pages to complete the explanation sentences in the table.
2. Use the Exam Tip on page 75 to write some explanation paragraphs.

Factors	Explanation – Why was this factor important?
The role of individuals	Fleming deserves credit for the initial discovery. Florey and Chain were important because …
Chance	Fleming left a pile of petri dishes when he …
Science and technology	Without the pharmaceutical industry, it would not have been possible to …
Warfare	The First World War motivated Fleming to start his research. The Second World War …
Government	The American government provided the funds for …
Communication	Florey and Chain read …

Florey and Chain

In 1938, Howard Florey and Ernst Chain were working together at Oxford University, researching how germs could be killed. They read Fleming's article on penicillin and realised that it could be very effective, so they tried to get funding from the British government to manufacture penicillin. They only got £25! Still Florey and Chain persevered. They tested penicillin on mice and discovered that it helped mice recover from infections. However, to treat one person they needed 3000 times as much penicillin as they had used to treat one mouse! So they began growing penicillin wherever they could, using hundreds of hospital bedpans, even though the metal was in demand for building Spitfire aeroplanes.

By 1941, Florey and Chain had enough penicillin to test it on one person. Their volunteer was Albert Alexander, a policeman. He had developed septicaemia (blood poisoning) from a tiny cut. The penicillin worked and Alexander began to recover. However, the penicillin ran out after five days. They were so desperate to continue the treatment that they extracted unused penicillin from the man's urine and reused it. Eventually, the penicillin ran out and the policeman became ill again and died. However, Florey and Chain had proved that penicillin worked and that it wasn't harmful to the patient. Their big question now was how to make enough of it?

Mass production

English factories were too busy making war supplies to help. So Florey went to America – at just the right time. In 1941, America was attacked by the Japanese at Pearl Harbour and entered the war. The American government realised the potential of penicillin for treating wounded soldiers and made interest-free loans to US companies to buy the expensive equipment needed for making penicillin. By 1944, there was enough to treat all the Allied wounded on D-Day in June – over 2.3 million doses.

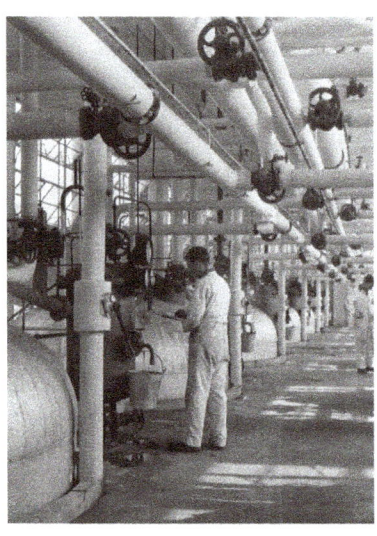

▲ **SOURCE 1** Tanks used to produce penicillin

Antibiotics for everyone

War led to the development of penicillin. It led to government investment and proved that penicillin could transform the treatment of many illnesses.

However, once the war ended in 1945, there was still a lot to do to make antibiotics available for the whole population.

- Pharmaceutical companies paid for researchers to discover and trial other antibiotics.
- Scientific techniques and technological equipment were improved to enable this work.
- After 1948, the government-funded NHS provided antibiotics free of charge.
- Scientists and doctors communicated their research so they could learn from each other.

The development of antibiotics transformed medicine. Before antibiotics, pneumonia, meningitis and similar infections often killed people. Afterwards, they were much more likely to survive.

Fleming's discovery set off a chain of events that saved millions of lives.

Exam Tip

Develop your answers to prove the importance of factors

1. Read the explanation paragraph below and the notes around it.
2. Finish the paragraph off.
3. Add another paragraph where you aim to prove that another factor played a crucial role in the development of penicillin.

The first sentence makes the argument clear – the factor was 'essential'.

The word 'without' signals where the answer becomes a developed explanation.

The fourth sentence provides an explanation of why the role of the drug companies was essential.

> Science and technology played an **essential** role in the development of penicillin. The pharmaceutical industry developed techniques to mass produce penicillin using expensive equipment. **Without** the use of the facilities shown in Source 1, penicillin could not have been produced in large enough quantities to save the lives of thousands of people. **Before** the involvement of the drug companies, Florey and Chain were struggling to produce enough penicillin to save just one person's life. **In 1941**, the penicillin they were producing to treat a policeman ran out and the patient died. Moreover, improved microscopes **made it possible for** Fleming to …

Two pieces of evidence have been used to support this argument (the role of the pharmaceutical industry and the importance of microscopes).

A precise example is provided to further support the argument.

Summarise

Here is a visual summary of the penicillin story. Penicillin made Fleming **FAMOUS**.

Fleming … discovers first …
Antibiotic … made from …
Mould … developed into penicillin by …
Others … Chain & Florey, who travelled to …
USA … to raise funds for use on …
Soldiers … in the Second World War.

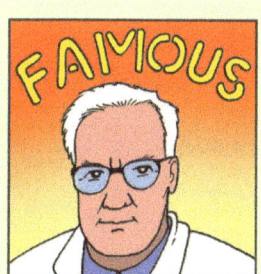

Turn this into your own memory aid by adding your own pictures for each stage. Keep it simple – do not spend a long time on your drawings. The important thing is that they are memorable to you, not that they are brilliant artwork.

10.3 The development of the pharmaceutical industry, new treatments and new diseases

Research & Record

How far has medicine progressed in the last 100 years?

The Germ Theory led to new methods of treating disease which significantly increased life expectancy in Britain. However, the last 100 years has also seen new problems.

Use the information on these two pages to draw up two lists like this.

- Areas where medicine has progressed
- New threats or challenges that remain

Pharmaceutical companies have competed to make more effective drugs ...

During the twentieth century, British companies such as Beechams became worldwide businesses, manufacturing drugs. They:

- invested in research and development (including employing scientists) and did careful experiments to look for better remedies
- used industrial technology to make huge quantities of each remedy.

Drug manufacture became big business. Drug companies could make a lot of money, save many lives and reduce suffering if they discovered an effective drug.

Case study: aspirin

Aspirin comes from willow bark and has been used as a medicine for centuries, although no one knew why it worked.

Developments in science enabled scientists to identify the exact chemical in willow bark that was beneficial. It was then manufactured in huge quantities. In the 1970s, researchers found that aspirin also helped to thin the blood and could help to prevent blood clots from forming. More recent research has shown that low doses of aspirin can reduce the risk of heart attack.

... and the discovery of DNA has uncovered the genetic causes of disease ...

Following the discovery that germs cause disease, for nearly 100 years, all the scientific focus was on illness caused by bacteria.

However, many illnesses have genetic causes – they are inherited in the genes. These include Alzheimer's disease, diabetes, Parkinson's disease and some forms of cancer.

Until the 1950s, these diseases were untreatable. This began to change in 1953, when the work of Rosalind Franklin enabled **Francis Crick and James Watson** to discover the structure of human DNA and how it passes from parents to their children.

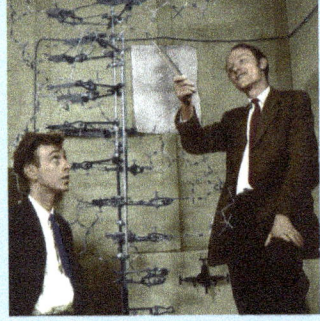

In the 1990s, the Human Genome Project, a worldwide project, began working out exactly how each part of human DNA affects the human body. This information has allowed scientists to find ways of treating specific genetic illnesses. For example, researchers have used computers to predict how cancer can evolve in individual patients. This should help doctors decide the most effective form of treatment for each individual patient and so boost their chances of survival.

... but, the fight against disease is not straightforward

Thalidomide

In the late 1950s, **thalidomide** was introduced as a 'safe' sleeping tablet. It was later given to women to reduce morning sickness during pregnancy. However, this drug had not been fully tested and led to children being born with severely deformed limbs.

Thalidomide was banned in 1961, but, by then, around 10,000 children worldwide had already been affected. Since then, research on thalidomide has continued and, in a different form, has been shown to help people with blood cancer and leprosy. The impact of thalidomide led to much more thorough testing of drugs before use.

Antibiotic resistance

Since the development of penicillin, new, stronger antibiotics have been produced. They have saved millions of lives (an estimated 200 million lives in 70 years).

However, within just a few decades of antibiotics being introduced, some bacteria began to develop immunity to the drugs. They have been labelled **'superbugs'**. MRSA is one example – it can resist science's efforts to kill it, either with antiseptics or antibiotics.

Overuse of antibiotics has made them less effective. This has become a major concern. In 2014, the World Health Organisation warned of a 'post-antibiotic era' in which common infections could once again kill because antibiotics simply no longer work.

New diseases – AIDS

New diseases have appeared. In 1982, doctors recognised a new illness, AIDS, which destroys the body's immunity to other diseases, leaving those with the illness much more vulnerable to infections and other diseases, such as cancer.

AIDS is transmitted through sexual fluids and blood. More than 40 million people worldwide have died of AIDS-related illnesses. A cure or effective vaccine has yet to be found.

However, in the 1990s, treatments such as HAART (highly active anti-retroviral therapy) were introduced that helped to improve long-term survival rates.

Alternative treatments

Drug treatments have been a big part of making us healthier, but there are some people who think that pharmaceutical companies are now part of the health problem – not the solution. Our response to any illness is 'must find the wonder drug', yet the solution to modern conditions can be found in other ways, called **alternative treatments**.

Lifestyle remedies

Doctors are now keenly aware that the biggest medical problems facing people in Britain are not infectious or genetic diseases, but the choices people make and the way they live their lives. For example:

- **Mental health problems** caused by not enough sleep and stressful working and home lives cause thousands of deaths each year.
- **Breathing difficulties caused** by polluted air put hundreds of thousands of people at risk each year.
- **Obesity** caused by people eating too much of the wrong kinds of food and exercising too little is now a leading cause of death, particularly among men.

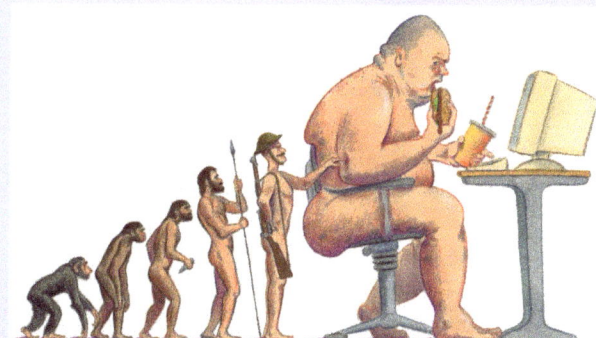

▲ A cartoonist's comment on the effect of a modern lifestyle

Traditional remedies

- **Acupuncture** has been used in China for 4000 years. It involves inserting fine needles at pressure points on the body to release blocked energy. It is used both to treat disease and as a painkiller during surgery.
- Many health shops sell '**herbal remedies**' made from plants and animal substances which have been used in medicine for centuries.

Topic 11: The impact of war and technology on surgery

11.1 The impact of the First and Second World Wars on surgery

Research & Record

How were the problems faced by surgeons during the two world wars overcome?

In wartime, doctors face extreme problems which need rapid solutions. Use a table like this to record the solutions that were developed.

Problem	Solution
Deep infections – bullets carried bacteria deep inside the body.	
Foreign bodies – it was hard to locate bullets and shrapnel deep inside the body.	
Disfiguring injuries could be caused by bullets or shell damage.	
Blood loss – many men died from blood loss even when the wound itself was not fatal.	

1 X-rays

In 1895, a German scientist, Wilhelm Röntgen, found that **X-rays** could pass through paper, wood and flesh – but not bone. Within months, the first X-ray machines were being used in hospitals to identify diseases and broken bones. However, it was the First World War that saw the technology being widely used.

Many casualties had bullets or shrapnel embedded deep in their body. X-rays helped surgeons find these objects quickly and remove them more easily and completely. This, in turn, reduced infection.

By 1916, all the major British army hospitals were using X-rays and ambulances fitted with X-ray equipment were being used close to the front line.

2 Improved antiseptic techniques

Surgeons experimented with new ways to prevent infection in wounds. For example, two doctors devised a system of tubes (the Carrel–Dakin method) which kept a chemical solution continually flowing through the wound to fight infection. Continuous use was more effective than a one-off treatment. As a result, fewer amputations led to infection.

3 Blood transfusions and blood banks

In the nineteenth century, the problems of infection and pain had been solved, but blood loss remained a major problem. This was greatly helped by developments before and during the First World War.

The discovery of blood groups

Blood transfusions had been attempted in the 1800s. Sometimes it worked; mostly, it did not. Nobody knew why. Then, in 1901, **Karl Landsteiner** discovered blood groups – that blood of one group cannot be mixed with blood of a different group. After this, blood transfusions became possible, as long as the patient and the donor were of the same blood group and in the same place.

Discovering how to handle blood

When doctors tried to store or transport blood, it clotted and could not be used. This problem was solved during the First World War.

- Firstly, sodium citrate was added to prevent the blood from clotting.
- Later in the war, scientists discovered how to separate and store the blood cells from the plasma and keep them in a 'blood bank' for future use.

Methods of storing blood continued to improve in the Second World War. Transfusions saved thousands of lives.

4 Plastic surgery

Plastic surgery had been carried out centuries earlier but it was limited by the danger of infection and pain. With these two problems solved, it paved the way for surgeons to repair some of the terrible wounds caused in war by bullets and shrapnel.

Improvements in the First World War

Surgeons carried out over 11,000 plastic surgery operations, increasing their experience and learning from each other. By November 1915, seven hospitals in France had specialist departments for dealing with wounds needing plastic surgery, particularly to the face and head.

Surgeons developed new techniques using jaw splints, wiring and metal plates as 'replacement' cheeks. Another major improvement was the use of skin grafts, taking skin from another part of the patient's body and grafting it on to the area of the wound.

Harold Gillies, a New Zealand surgeon, serving in France, persuaded the army's chief surgeon that a specialist facial injury care unit was needed in England for the wounded. In 1917, The Queen's Hospital was opened in Kent, specialising in repairing facial injuries.

Improvements in the Second World War

In the Second World War, fighting technology had moved on. Soldiers fought in aircraft and tanks rather than by charging at the enemy. Burns were a common injury in this type of warfare and plastic surgeons became expert in repairing burn damage.

Archibald McIndoe (Consultant in Plastic Surgery to the RAF) carried out 4000 operations on burns. He used skin grafts to reconstruct airmen's faces and hands. He also helped his patients psychologically to deal with the great changes in their appearance and the horrors they had been through. He even helped some of his patients financially to start life again as civilians. His patients were devoted to him, setting up The Guinea Pig Club, open to all those he treated.

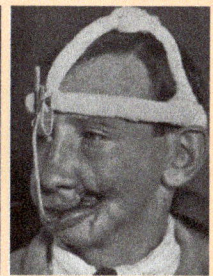
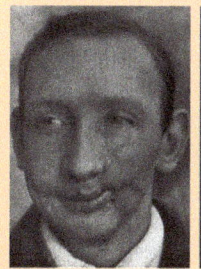
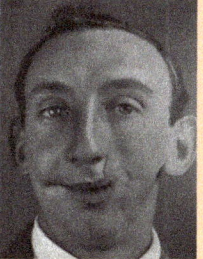

▲ **SOURCE 1** Photographs showing the reconstruction of a soldier's face, from a 1920 report by Harold Gillies

Summarise

Can you remember what these visuals help you remember?

1 **PILE**

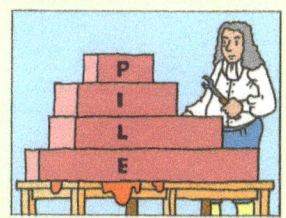

2 **AAA**

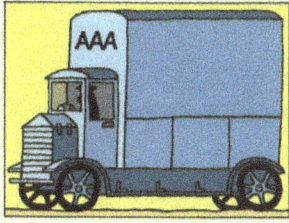

3 Use the BBB memory aid below to help you remember how the problem of blood loss was solved during the twentieth century. Explain how each of these Bs helped to overcome the problem of blood loss.

Dealing with blood loss = 3Bs

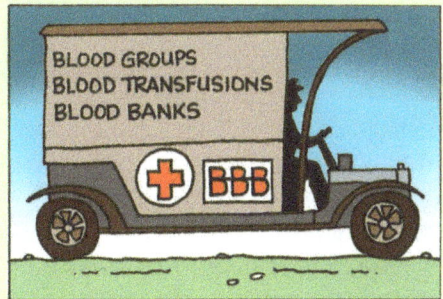

11.2 Modern surgical methods

Research & Record

How has better science and technology improved modern surgery?

Use the information boxes on pages 80 and 81 to complete a table like this to record how science and technology has improved each area of surgery. The table has been started with information from the previous two pages.

Improvements in surgery	How has better science and technology led to improvements?
Antiseptics	The Carrel–Dakin method kept a chemical solution flowing through the wound to fight infection.
Treating broken bones	X-ray machines helped surgeons locate injuries and illnesses.
Blood transfusions	Sodium citrate stopped blood clotting when it was stored. This helped in the development of blood banks.
Anaesthetics	
Diagnosis and treatment of cancers	
Surgery (open-heart, transplant and keyhole)	

1 Injected anaesthetics

In the 1800s, anaesthetics were inhaled through the nose and mouth. This made it hard to control the dosage. Surgeons erred on the side of caution for fear of killing their patients, so still tended to operate as fast as they could.

In the 1930s, Helmuth Wesse developed anaesthetics that could be injected into the blood stream. This allowed more precise dosage and, therefore, improved safety. This permitted longer operations. Nowadays, local anaesthetics are so effective that patients can even have major operations, such as hip-replacements, without going to sleep at all.

2 Radiation therapy and chemotherapy

Radiation therapy (or radiotherapy as it is also called) developed from Röntgen's discovery of X-rays.

Marie Curie, a Polish scientist, played a very important role. While she was researching X-rays with her husband, Pierre, they noticed that the skin on their hands was burned by the material they were handling. This led to the discovery of radium, which has been used ever since to diagnose and to treat cancers. Their research was the beginning of the modern treatment of cancers. Sadly, Marie Curie herself died of leukaemia, caused by the radioactive material she used in her research.

Radiotherapy aims to kill the cancer cells using beams of radiation. Techniques have improved to target cancers more precisely.

Since the 1970s, **chemotherapy** has been used if cancer has developed so far that surgery and radiotherapy are not successful. Chemotherapy involves using particularly powerful chemicals to attack the cancer cells, although it can have significant side effects because healthy cells are killed too.

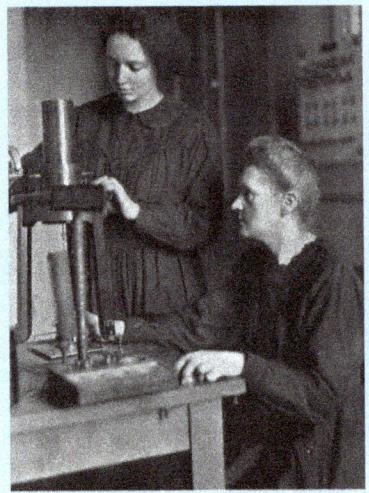

▼ SOURCE 1 Marie Curie (1867–1934), with her daughter in 1920. She is the only woman to have won two Nobel Prizes, for her work on X-rays and on radium

3 Open-heart surgery

Improvements in technology have led to dramatic advances in heart surgery. The heart/lung machine was designed to bypass the heart and maintain blood circulation while surgery is carried out on the stopped heart. This enabled surgeons to replace diseased valves or repair defects in the walls between the chambers of the heart. By the 1970s, heart bypasses had become common and heart surgery quite routine.

4 Transplant surgery

The first heart **transplant** was carried out in South Africa in 1967. Other organs had been transplanted before then (kidneys in 1954 and a liver in 1963) and, since then, even more ambitious transplants have been carried out, including the first bone marrow transplant in 1980, and the first heart and lung transplant in 1982.

All transplants depend on technical skill and many other discoveries. For example, before transplants could work, scientists had to first discover drugs to stop the patient's body rejecting their new replacement organs.

5 Keyhole surgery

Major surgery used to mean surgeons making large cuts into the body. Nowadays, large incisions are avoided as often as possible. Instead '**keyhole surgery**' allows surgeons to work through a tiny hole to carry out complex operations.

This is possible because of miniaturisation – all the surgeon's tools are inside a small instrument called an **endoscope** which is controlled by the surgeon from outside using miniature cameras, fibre-optic cables and computers.

6 Scanning machines

X-rays made it possible to see inside the body without surgery. Modern scanners built on that foundation.

CT scanners can take thousands of X-ray readings in a second. As the patient passes through a hoop-shaped machine, the scanner rotates around the frame, sending and detecting beams of x-rays through the body. This produces a 3D image. This is especially useful in examining the internal structure of lungs, which cannot be seen clearly using simple radiography.

Magnetic resonance imaging (MRI) uses magnets and radio waves rather than X-Rays. It can detect cancer cells and is particularly useful when examining the brain and nerves.

Ultrasound scanners can assess the blood flow in veins and arteries.

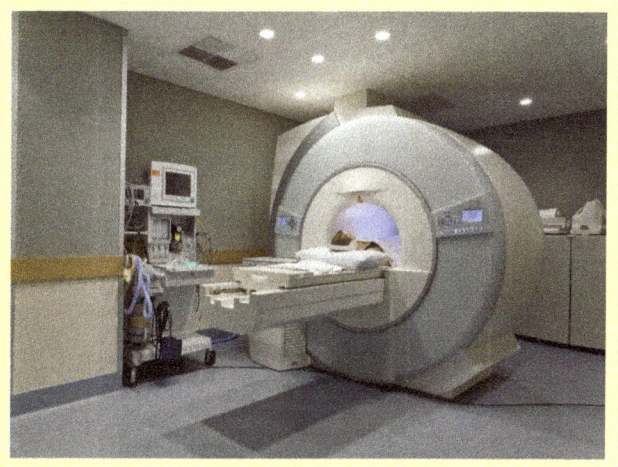

7 Robotic surgery

Surgeons can now use robots to carry out some operations. Robots can be more precise and controlled than human surgeons. Nanobots (tiny specialised robots less than a millimetre long) can perform tasks such as clearing arteries.

Summarise

Use the memory aid **PLASTIC** to help you remember the key improvements in surgery since 1900. Complete this memory aid by adding brief explanations and/or examples to each key improvement.

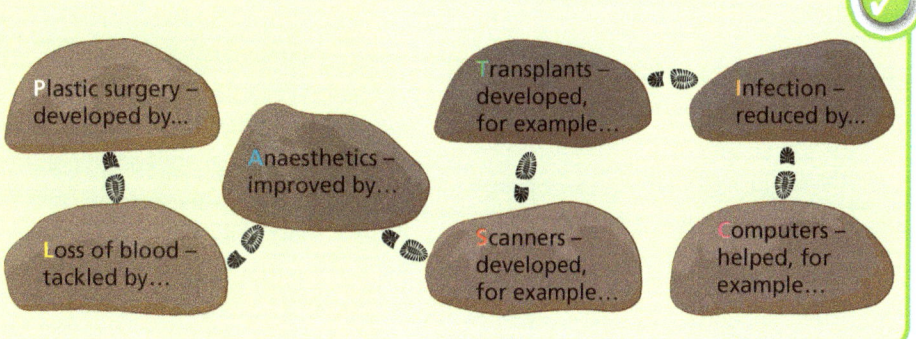

11.2 Modern surgical methods

81

11.3 The factors behind improvements in surgery

> **Review**
>
> **Has science and technology been the main influence on the development of surgery?**
>
> Science and technology has clearly had a major influence on the development of modern surgery, but was this the case for other periods of history? Even when we consider modern medicine, were other factors, such as the role of war or the government, more important?
>
> 1 Look at the summary of how surgery has developed since 1000 below. For each period:
>   a Identify at least one individual who played an important role in improving surgery. Look at the yellow box below (left) for a reminder of the key individuals.
>   b Identify at least two other factors that you think influenced surgery in this period. Make sure that you can explain how this factor played a role.
> 2 Use your research notes to attempt the exam practice Question 4 on page 83.

Factor: INDIVIDUALS
- Joseph Lister
- Archibald McIndoe
- Guy de Chauliac
- Karl Landsteiner
- Harold Gillies
- Ambroise Paré
- James Simpson

Summary: How has surgery developed?	
c1000–1500	• Basic surgery on visible wounds and tumours, splints for fractured bones • Some improvements made by battlefield surgeons (e.g. metal forceps) • Simple anaesthetics made from plants • Honey, wine and vinegar used as antiseptics • Cauterisation used to stop blood loss
c1500–1800	• Improved treatment of gunshot wounds (e.g. use of bandages and ointments rather than boiling oil) • Use of ligatures to stop bleeding (although cauterisation still widely used) • Simple anaesthetics and antiseptics • First blood transfusions attempted, but no understanding of blood groups • Development of artificial limbs
c1800–1900	• Longer and more complex surgery made possible by development of ways to reduce pain and stop infection • Anaesthetics introduced (e.g. ether and chloroform) • Carbolic acid spray introduced as an effective antiseptic • The start of aseptic surgery (e.g. surgeons wear masks, gowns and rubber gloves, sterilised surgical equipment) • Status of surgeons improved – they become more respected as a profession
c1900–present	• Discovery of blood groups and the development of ways to store blood leads to blood banks for blood transfusions • Further improvements in antiseptics (e.g. Carrel–Dakin method) and anaesthetics (e.g. local anaesthetics) • Introduction of new equipment to help with diagnosis and operations (e.g. X-rays, body scanners, ECGs) • Transplant surgery • Keyhole surgery

Apply ▶ Exam Practice

Question 4 style

How far has science and technology been the main factor in the development of surgery in Britain? **(16 marks)**

Exam Tips

Question 4 – the role of factors

1. **Weigh** the importance of science and technology against **two other factors**. Write one paragraph explaining how each factor played an important role.
2. **Select** examples to support the points you make from a **range of time periods**. Aim to refer to **all four time periods** in your answer.
3. **Evaluate** the importance of each factor **using clear criteria**. Demonstrate complex thinking. Think carefully about:

   a. LENGTH OF TIME – Did it play an important role across all four time periods?

   b. SCALE OF IMPACT – How important was the role played in each time period? Was it crucial or essential to the developments that took place? Or did it speed up changes that were already taking place (playing more of a facilitating or contributory role)?

   c. LINKS TO OTHER FACTORS – Did it influence other factors? For example:

   Link 1 WARFARE → provided an opportunity for → INDIVIDUALS such as Paré, Gillies and McIndoe to develop new techniques.

   Link 2 SCIENCE & TECHNOLOGY → gave a better understanding of chemicals such as chloroform so → INDIVIDUALS such as Simpson and Lister could develop anaesthetics and antiseptics.

4. Reach a **clear conclusion**. Make sure you directly address the question. Focus on the phrases 'how far' and 'main factor' that appear in the question. **How far** was science and technology more important than any other factor in the development of surgery? To a large extent? To some extent? Was it the **main factor**? Or did other factors have a larger impact over a longer period of time?

Apply ▶ Exam Practice

Question 2 style

Explain the significance of the work of James Simpson in the development of surgery. **(8 marks)**

Question 3 style

Explain two ways in which medieval surgery and surgery at the time of Paré were similar. Explain your answer with reference to both time periods. **(8 marks)**

Exam Tips

Think long-term as well as short-term impact. Use what you have learnt about anaesthetics (page 62) and modern surgery (Topic 11) to show how anaesthetics were developed and are still important today.

Make two direct comparisons. Base each of your paragraphs around a theme. Use your PILE memory aid. For example, you could compare how surgeons dealt with two of these problems:

- pain
- infection
- blood loss.

Topic 12: Modern public health

12.1 The Liberal social reforms

Research & Record

Who influenced and who benefited from the Liberal social reforms of 1906–14?

Use pages 84 and 85 to fill in a copy of the bingo card.

Liberal social reforms bingo		
What percentage of recruits were rejected during the Boer War because they were unfit?	**At what age** could people get an Old Age Pension after 1908?	**Which group** of people benefited from the National Insurance Act after 1911?
Give 2 ways that Rowntree influenced the actions of the Liberal government.	**Give 2 examples** of things taught in medical schools for mothers.	**Which 2 groups** paid into the National Insurance scheme, apart from workers?
Give 3 ways in which Booth influenced the actions of the Liberal government.	**Give 3 examples** of how young children benefited from Liberal social reforms.	**List 3 groups** of people who did not benefit from the National Insurance Act.

Demands for reform

By 1900, life expectancy was starting to rise. It had reached 46 for men and 50 for women. Towns were cleaner. Public health facilities were beginning to improve. But the key words here are 'starting to' and 'beginning to'.

The problem of poverty

Many people still experienced major health problems, partly because of dirt but even more because of poverty. The government gave no help to sick, unemployed or older people. Those who could not get help from friends and relatives or charities had to go into a workhouse, run by the local council. The infant death rate (see Source 1) was still very high. One in seven babies died before they reached their first birthday!

Researchers such as Charles Booth and Seebohm Rowntree published reports which showed just how poor many people were and also showed the links between poverty and ill-health.

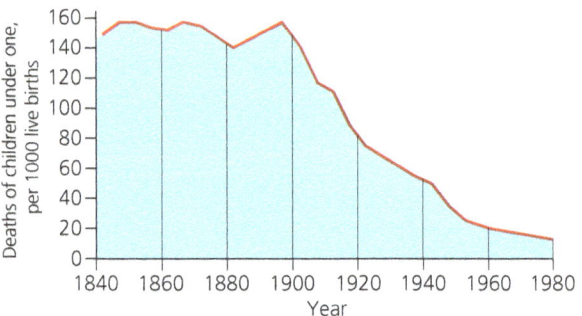

▲ **SOURCE 1** The death rate of children under one year old, 1840–1980. Today, it is remarkable how much infant mortality rates have fallen since the early twentieth century

Probably even more shocking to the government was the finding from medical inspections when they tried to raise an army to fight the Boer War. An incredible 38 per cent of all potential recruits were unfit to serve on medical grounds. Governments might not have thought solving the problem of poverty was their job – but having a strong army was!

The Liberal reforms, 1906–14

Who influenced them?

Seebohm Rowntree
The Rowntrees owned a famous chocolate factory in York. In 1901, Seebohm Rowntree published a study of living conditions in York, showing that more than a quarter of the people in York were living in poverty and that this was seriously harming their health. Rowntree's report deeply influenced people within the Liberal government that came into power in 1906.

Charles Booth
Booth was a businessman who paid for research into poverty in the East End of London between 1889 and 1903. He also spent weeks living in the area himself. He discovered that 35 per cent of people were living in poverty – far more than had been claimed. Booth argued that government should take responsibility for caring for people in poverty. One of his suggestions was an old-age pension.

David Lloyd George

Lloyd George was a brilliant, persuasive speaker, determined to improve the lives of ordinary people and was a friend of Rowntree. He was Chancellor of the Exchequer (deciding on how the government raises and spends its money) in the Liberal government. He increased the taxes paid by the rich to pay for the reforms listed below (left).

In 1906, a new Liberal government was elected by a vast majority. Their election campaign had included promises to tackle poverty – and over the next six years they delivered. These reforms may seem ordinary today, but a hundred years ago they were revolutionary.

- **1906** Free school meals for school children.
- **1907** All births had to be reported to the local Medical Officer. A health visitor then visited each mother to make sure she knew how to protect her baby's health. Free medical checks for school children.
- **1908** Old-age pensions introduced for people over 70 who did not have enough money to live on.
- **1909** New laws enforced higher standards of house building.
- **1911** National Insurance Act provided help for sick people (see panel).
- **1912** Clinics set up to provide free medical treatment for children in school.

National Insurance Act, 1911
This was one of the greatest changes introduced by the Liberal government. It gave workers medical help and sick pay if they could not work through illness. Until then, workers who fell ill had a choice: carry on working although they were ill, or not work and get no pay, which usually meant they could not afford medical help either.

The **National Insurance** scheme required workers, their employer and the government to pay into a sickness fund. (The government contributed 2d per week, the employer 3d and the worker 4d). When workers fell ill and were unable to work, they received 10d a week for up to 26 weeks and free medical care. This was paid out of the sickness fund. It was a major step forward, although it only covered people in work, not their families. Most women and all children were excluded. So were unemployed people, older people and anyone who had a long-lasting illness.

Summarise

Lloyd George and the Liberal reforms … **OPENS** the door for further public health improvements:

Old age
Pensions
Education for mothers
National Insurance
School meals and medical checks

12.2 The impact of two world wars on public health, poverty and housing

Research & Record

How did the First and Second World Wars change attitudes towards public health?

1. Give at least two examples to support statements A and B below.

   A Housing was improved after the First World War. For example, …

   B In the 1930s, Britain still faced major public health problems. For example, …

2. Explain how each of the following factors played a role in establishing a National Health Service in 1948.
   a   The Second World War
   b   The role of individuals (William Beveridge and Aneurin Bevan)

'Homes fit for heroes': improvements in housing

During the First World War, Lloyd George had promised 'Homes fit for heroes' for the returning soldiers. Immediately after the war ended, the government introduced the 1919 Housing Act. This forced local councils to provide good homes for working people to rent. A quarter of a million new homes were built in the early 1920s. The Act also set standards for space, water supply and drainage for all new houses.

In the 1930s, many old, unhealthy slum houses were demolished and another 700,000 new houses were built.

'The Hungry Thirties': National Insurance under strain

In the 1930s, Britain suffered a severe economic depression. Unemployment rose to more than 3 million, causing widespread poverty. People struggled to find the money to buy food and to heat their homes. Only about half of the population was covered by National Insurance; children and those who did not work lost out. The National Insurance Scheme did not help unemployed people. Even those with a job faced problems. Employers reduced working hours and reduced wages, so even people in work fell behind on the payments which guaranteed them free medical help. The 1911 system was failing. The most worrying evidence came from towns where unemployment was high. Infant mortality was rising again.

▼ **SOURCE 1** From an interview with Kathleen Davys, one of a Birmingham family of 13 children growing up in the 1920s and 1930s. The local doctor charged sixpence for each visit

For headaches, we had vinegar and brown paper; for whooping cough we had camphorated oil rubbed on our chests or goose fat. For mumps we had stockings round our throats and measles we had tea stewed in the teapot by the fire – all different kinds of home cures. They thought they were better than going to the doctor. Well they couldn't afford the doctor.

The impact of the Second World War

The Second World War put a severe strain on the British people. It required sacrifices from everyone. 400,000 British soldiers died, but also 60,000 British civilians were killed in bombing raids. For six years, the country felt it was living on the edge. Yet it pulled through. After all these sacrifices, people wanted, and were prepared to work together and pay for, a better future.

War also opened some people's eyes to poverty – for example, children were evacuated from towns to the countryside and the middle-class families in rural areas were appalled at how unhealthy some evacuee children were.

It also set a new pattern of government help. During the war the government had to provide free health care to keep the country running and because of civilian casualties.

The Beveridge Report

In 1941, the national coalition government asked William Beveridge to write a report on what should be done to improve people's lives after the war. Beveridge had played a key part in creating the 1911 National Insurance Scheme, so could see how it could be improved.

In his report, he set out measures to slay the five giants of 'Squalor (poor housing), ignorance (bad education), want (poverty), idleness (unemployment) and disease (ill-health)'. His main recommendations were:

- A **national health service**, free to everyone and paid for from taxes. Doctors, nurses and other medical workers would become government employees, instead of charging sick people to pay their wages.
- **Universal national insurance**. Everyone in work would contribute out of their wages. This money would be used, by the government, to pay benefits (sick-pay, old-age pensions, unemployment pay, etc.) to everyone, whether they had been workers or not.

The Beveridge Report spelled out a cradle-to-grave **welfare state** and, understandably, was greeted with great enthusiasm. People queued to buy a copy. 600,000 copies were sold.

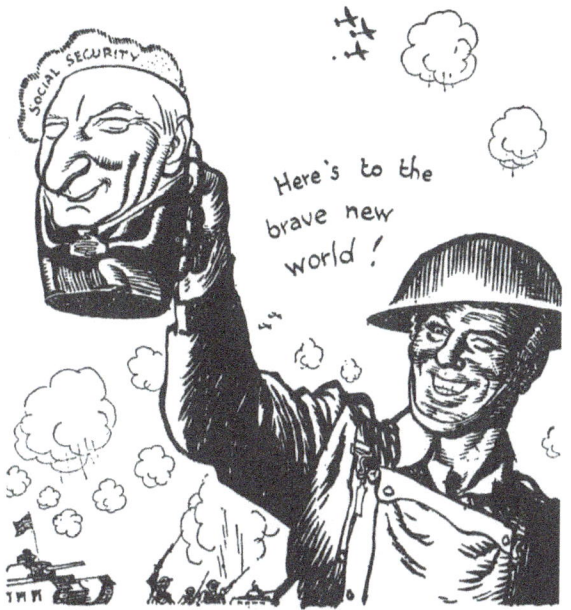

▲ **SOURCE 2** A cartoon from the *Daily Mail*, 2 December 1942, reporting the publication of the Beveridge Report. ('Beverage' was the similar word used at the time for a drink)

The role played by Bevan and the 1945–51 Labour Government

The Beveridge Report was only a report. He did not decide the law. Only the government could make that decision. So what to do in reaction to the Beveridge Report became a key issue in the post-war general election. The 1945 election was a vote on what kind of country people wanted Britain to be.

The Labour Party promised to establish a national health service. Their manifesto was called 'Let us face the future'. They won a landslide victory.

Their new Health Minister was Aneurin Bevan. He was an inspiring public speaker and determined to improve life for working people. Through his work for the miners' union, he had seen the problems caused by poverty and sickness. His speeches in favour of the NHS won support for Labour's plans.

In 1946, Bevan, introduced his plans to Parliament. He said that *'medical treatment should be made available to rich and poor alike in accordance with medical need and no other criteria'*.

As you will see, Bevan faced opposition but, in July 1948, the NHS was introduced, providing free medical services for everyone.

12.3 The creation and development of the National Health Service

Research & Record

What short-term impact did the NHS have on medicine in Britain?

Use the information below and a table like this one to collect evidence of how the NHS affected each area of medicine.

Area of medicine	Evidence of impact
Treatment	
Prevention	
Hospitals and health centres	
Training of doctors and nurses	

The changes introduced by the NHS

The NHS was introduced in July 1948. Now everyone could get free medical treatment. Until 1948, 8 million people had never seen a doctor because they could not afford to do so. The diagram shows the range of services provided by the NHS.

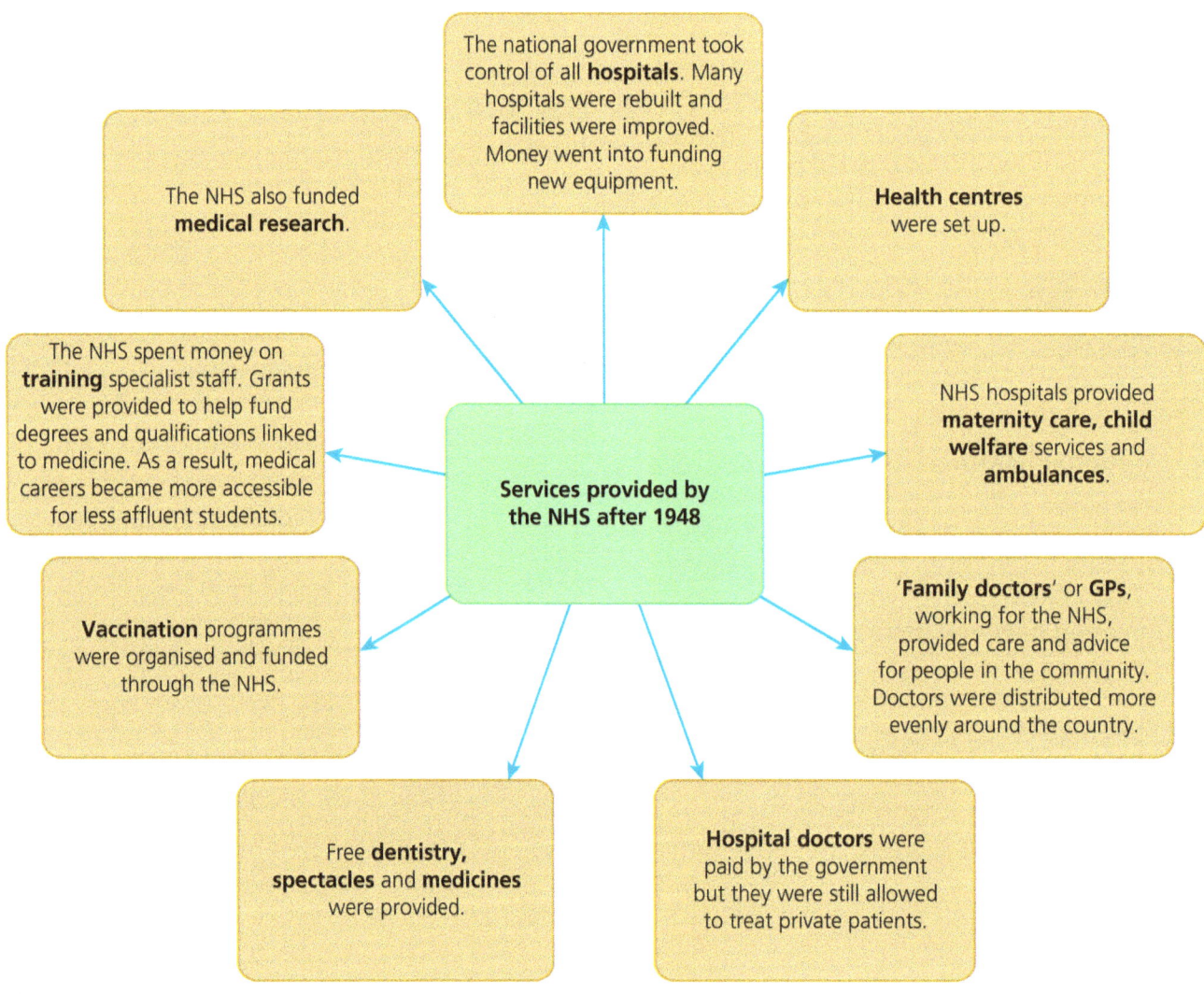

Services provided by the NHS after 1948:

- The national government took control of all **hospitals**. Many hospitals were rebuilt and facilities were improved. Money went into funding new equipment.
- The NHS also funded **medical research**.
- **Health centres** were set up.
- The NHS spent money on **training** specialist staff. Grants were provided to help fund degrees and qualifications linked to medicine. As a result, medical careers became more accessible for less affluent students.
- NHS hospitals provided **maternity care, child welfare** services and **ambulances**.
- **Vaccination** programmes were organised and funded through the NHS.
- 'Family doctors' or **GPs**, working for the NHS, provided care and advice for people in the community. Doctors were distributed more evenly around the country.
- Free **dentistry, spectacles** and **medicines** were provided.
- **Hospital doctors** were paid by the government but they were still allowed to treat private patients.

Why was there opposition to the NHS?

Despite the general enthusiasm for Beveridge's report and the idea of creating a national health service, there was powerful opposition.

- The most important opposition came from doctors themselves. They feared they would lose their independence (see Source 1). They were also afraid that they would lose their freedom to treat private patients who paid fees. Some doctors made a lot of money as private consultants, treating rich patients who were willing to pay high fees to see the very best physicians. Bevan dealt with this opposition by agreeing that doctors could continue to treat patients privately and charge them fees, as well as working for the NHS.
- Some people believed that those living in poverty should not be helped. They thought that less affluent people would grow lazy if they were getting 'something for nothing' and this would make people less likely to bother working.
- Some local councils and charities did not want the government taking over control of their hospitals.

▼ **SOURCE 1** Two extracts from the *British Medical Journal*, the official journal of the medical profession

A If a National Health Service is set up then doctors will no longer be independent. They will instead be technicians controlled by civil servants and by men and women entirely ignorant of medical matters.

B If the Bill is passed, no patient or doctor will feel safe from interference by some government regulation. The minister's spies will be everywhere.

Apply ▶ Exam Practice

Question 1 style

Use Source 2 to practise answering source-based questions.

How useful is the source 2 to a historian studying reactions to Bevan's plans to establish the NHS? (8 marks)

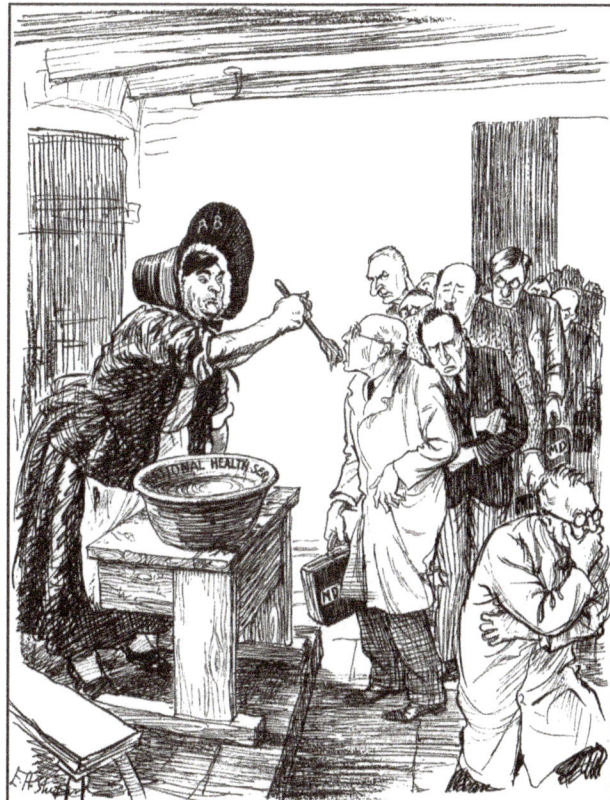

◀ **SOURCE 2** A cartoon published in 1948. The figure on the left is Bevan. The words in the bowl say 'National Health Service'. The doctors on the right are saying 'It all tastes awful'

12.4 Costs, choices and the issues of healthcare in the twenty-first century

Research & Record

How has the NHS changed since 1948 and what challenges does it face?

The NHS came into existence on 5 July 1948. It was the first time anywhere in the world that completely free healthcare was made available. Doctors, nurses, dentists and hospitals were brought together under one service.

Read pages 90 and 91.
1. Identify and explain the three main ways that the NHS has changed since 1948.
2. Identify and explain three challenges that the NHS faces in the twenty-first century.
3. Identify and explain three ways in which the NHS has helped to improve life expectancy in Britain since the Second World War.

The main changes to the NHS

1 Many more staff are employed

With 1.7 million people working for it, the NHS is the fifth largest employer in the world. This reflects how demand has increased.
- There are ten times as many doctors as there were in 1948.
- The number of nurses has trebled since 1948. Their role has become more specialised and it is now a degree-level profession.

2 Costs the country a lot more money

Since 1948, governments have had to invest more and more money in the NHS. Out-of-date hospitals have to be rebuilt to meet modern standards. In 2018, 30 pence in every pound spent by the government on public services went to the NHS. The amount spent on health is now 12 times more than it was when the NHS started (£12.9 bn in 1948, £149.2 bn in 2018) and costs are likely to carry on increasing. The more the government spends on health, the less it can spend on education, defence and housing.

3 Some patients are now charged for NHS services

In the early 1950s, the government struggled to keep up with the demand for free healthcare and to find the money to pay for it. Charges were introduced for prescriptions, dental work and spectacles.

4 Number of hospital beds cut

There are now far fewer beds. In 1948, there were 480,000 hospital beds; today there are just 120,000. The reason for this is that more healthcare is now provided in the community and patients spend less time in hospital. For example, when the NHS was established, women would often spend a week in hospital after giving birth. Today, they tend to leave hospital on the same day or the day after.

5 NHS now focuses on prevention as well as treatment

- **Lifestyle campaigns.** The deadly impact of illnesses such as cancer and heart disease has led to much greater efforts to persuade people to live healthier lives. Single-issue campaigns have focused on warning of the dangers of smoking and of lack of exercise or have promoted healthier diets.
- **Health checks.** In 1992, the government's 'Health of the Nation' initiative set the NHS targets to prevent and reduce deaths and illnesses in five major areas: heart disease, cancer, mental illness, HIV/AIDS and accidents. Everyone over the age of 40 can have a health check every five years, focusing on blood pressure, weight and cholesterol levels alongside lifestyle advice.

The impact of the NHS

1 Babies are less likely to die

Infant mortality (measured by deaths before the baby's first birthday) has improved dramatically (see page 84). The NHS has had a significant impact in this area. Most births now take place in a hospital, rather than at home. Hospitals can provide specialised support and equipment.

2 Immunisation campaigns have eradicated some illnesses

There is now a comprehensive vaccine programme in childhood with immunisations covering everything from meningitis and mumps to whooping cough. This has saved lives and increased life expectancy.

The introduction of the polio vaccine in the 1950s is a perfect example of this. Before this programme, there could be as many as 8,000 cases of polio in Britain in a year, but once people started getting immunised the numbers dropped quickly. There has not been a single case of polio in Britain since the 1980s.

3 People live longer

People now live 13 years longer than they did in 1948. (In 1948, life expectancy for a man was 65.9 years and for a woman 70.3 years. In 2018, these figures have risen to 79.5 years and 83.1 years respectively.)

Better access to healthcare has played a significant role. But it is also worth noting that in the 70 years before the creation of the NHS, life expectancy actually increased at a faster rate.

Two key factors in improving life expectancy at that stage, before the NHS, were access to clean water and the construction of sewers.

4 As life expectancy has increased, the causes of deaths have changed

Improved healthcare and vaccination programmes mean infectious diseases, heart attacks and strokes no longer kill as many people as they once did. Instead, people are more likely to be living with long-term conditions for which there are no cures. One example is dementia.

Cause of death	1948	2018
Heart disease	28.8%	15.7%
Stroke	11.2%	6.2%
Tuberculosis	4.7%	0.0%
Cancer	16.8%	27.8%
Diabetes	0.8%	1.1%
Dementia	2.6%	10.5%

Summarise

1. Can you remember why the changes introduced by the Liberal government between 1906 and 1914 were important? Use the **OPENS** memory aid to help you.
2. Complete the memory aid below. Explain each of the phrases on the NHS ambulance. Why was the introduction of the NHS so significant?

The National Health Service **TURNED** a corner for the people's health in Britain.

Training and research

Universal medicine (treatment and prevention) for all

Resources and equipment

New hospitals and health centres

Education – health campaigns

Doctors and GPs available to all

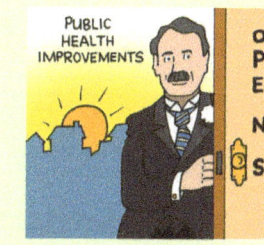
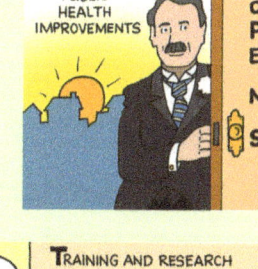

12.4 Costs, choices and the issues of healthcare in the 21st century

12.5 Twentieth century period review

Review

Which factor had the greatest impact on life expectancy?

The graph shows life expectancy for men and women through history.

Complete the factor cards below to explain how:
a science and technology
b government
c warfare

have contributed to this rise in life expectancy.

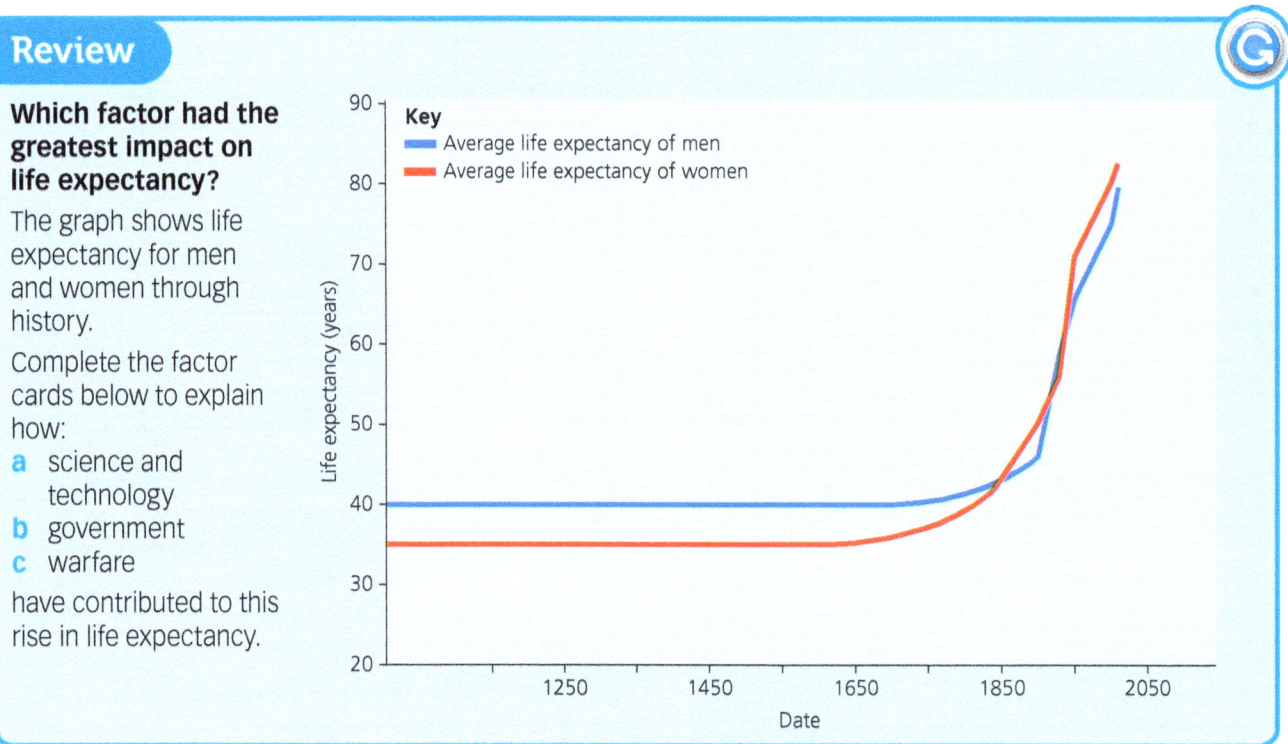

Key
— Average life expectancy of men
— Average life expectancy of women

Factor 1: Science and technology

Has improved diagnosis …
(e.g. X-rays or MRI)

Has made surgery more ambitious …
(e.g. keyhole surgery, transplant surgery)

Has revolutionised treatments …
(e.g. antibiotics)

Has prevented disease …
(e.g. vaccines)

Factor 2: Government

Has funded the NHS …
(e.g. paid for new technology in hospitals to diagnose and treat illness)

Has passed laws to …
(e.g. reduce air pollution or improve food safety to reduce food poisoning)

Has educated people …
(e.g. encouraging healthy lifestyles – warnings on cigarette packets)

Factor 3: Warfare

Led to improvements in surgery …
(e.g. First World War – blood transfusion)

Led to the development of penicillin …
In the First World War, Alexander Fleming …
During the Second World War …

Led to improvements in public health …
The Boer War influenced …
During the Second World War …

Apply ▶ Exam practice

Here is a full set of exam-style questions covering the whole course. Use the Exam Tips throughout the book to help you answer each type of question.

Question 1

Study Source A. How useful is Source A to a historian studying modern public health? (8 marks)

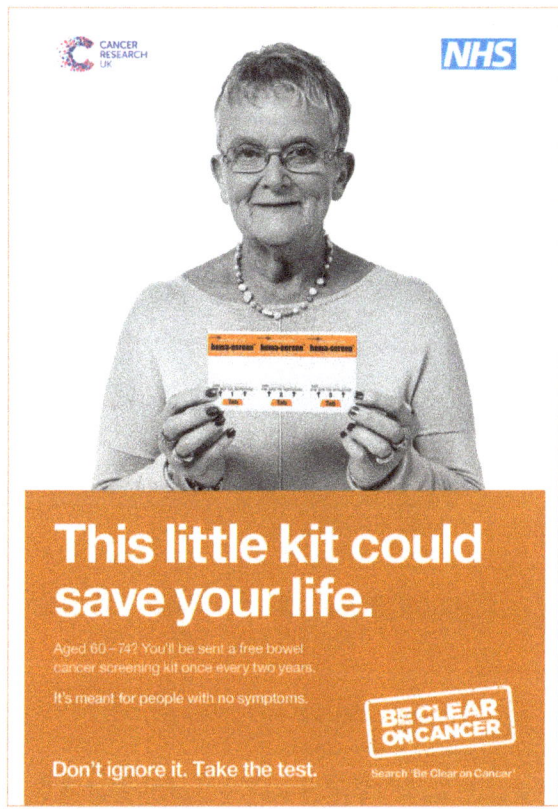

▲ **SOURCE A** This poster was part of a national advertising campaign by Cancer Research UK to get people to join the NHS Bowel Cancer Screening Programme. The campaign began in 2017 and aimed to diagnose bowel cancer earlier and so give patients a much better chance of survival

Question 2

Explain the significance of the NHS in the development of modern medicine. (8 marks)

Question 3

Explain two ways in which the treatment of disease in the nineteenth century and the treatment of disease by the end of the twentieth century were different. Explain your answer with reference to both time periods. (8 marks)

Question 4

How far has the government been the main factor in the development of public health in Britain since medieval times? Explain your answer with reference to government and other factors. (16 marks)

GLOSSARY

> **Revision Tip**
>
> Regularly test your understanding of the key terms in the glossary. You can do this in a number of ways:
>
> 1. Look at key terms in the list below which are marked in **BLUE**. Link each term to one of the individuals in the bingo card below. Make sure you can explain the link.
>
> | Health and the People Bingo | | | |
> |---|---|---|---|
> | Pasteur | Lister | Simpson | Galen |
> | Bazalgette | Snow | Lloyd-George | Bevan |
> | Vesalius | Paré | Jenner | Ehrlich |
> | Fleming | Curie | Harvey | Rowntree |
>
> 2. Look at the 10 words marked in **RED**. Place each word in one of the time periods below:
>
> | Medieval, c1000–1500 | Renaissance and Early Modern, c1500–1800 | Nineteenth century, 1800–1900 | Modern period, 1900–today |
> |---|---|---|---|
>
> 3. For all the other key words below, attempt both of these activities:
>   a. Ask someone to read out a definition (without the word) and see if you can guess the key term.
>   b. Ask someone to read out a key term and see if you can explain to them what the term means. If possible, aim to give an example to support your definition.

ALTERNATIVE TREATMENTS a way of treating an illness that is not based on mainstream, scientific medicine

AMPUTATION the removal of a limb by surgery

AMULET a charm that the wearer believes gives protection from disease

ANAESTHETIC a drug or drugs given to produce unconsciousness before and during surgery

ANATOMY the science of understanding the structure and make-up of the body

ANTIBIOTICS a group of drugs used to treat infections caused by bacteria, e.g. penicillin

ANTISEPTICS chemicals used to destroy bacteria and prevent infection

ARTERIES blood vessels that carry blood away from the heart

ASEPTIC SURGERY the performance of an operation under completely sterile conditions (free of all living micro-organisms)

ASTROLOGY the study of the planets and how they might influence the lives of people

BARBER SURGEON medieval barber who also performed surgery and dentistry

BEVERIDGE REPORT a report that outlined what should be done to improve people's lives after the Second World War. It recommended the setting up of the NHS.

BEZOAR STONE a ball of indigestible material found in goats' stomachs

BLACK DEATH a phrase used in the Middle Ages to describe bubonic plague. (The 'blackness' was caused by bleeding under the skin. Over 50 per cent of all cases were fatal)

BLEEDING the treatment of opening a vein or applying leeches to draw blood from the patient

BUBOES black swellings in the armpits and groin that were symptoms of the Black Death

CARBOLIC SPRAY used during surgical operations to kill germs in the air around the operating table

CAUTERISE using a hot iron to burn body tissue. This seals a wound and stops bleeding

CESSPOOL/CESSPIT a place for collecting and storing sewage

CHEMOTHERAPY treatment of a disease such as cancer by the use of chemicals

CHOLERA an infection that causes severe watery diarrhoea (it often results from drinking dirty water)

CHLOROFORM a liquid whose vapour acts as an anaesthetic and produces unconsciousness

'CURE-ALLS' a medicine usually sold for a profit. In the nineteenth century they were often made from a mix of ingredients that had no medical benefits

DISSECTION the cutting up and examination of a body

DNA deoxyribonucleic acid, the molecule that genes are made of. *See also* gene

DYSENTERY a severe infection causing frequent, fluid bowel movements

EPIDEMIC a sudden, widespread appearance of an infectious disease

ENDOSCOPE an instrument used to view inside the body

GENE part of a cell that determines how our bodies look and work. Genes are passed from parents to children

GERM a micro-organism that causes disease

GERM THEORY the theory that germs cause disease, often by infection through the air

HERBAL REMEDY a medicine made up from a mixture of plants, often containing beneficial ingredients

HUMOURS the Ancient Greeks believed the body contained four humours of liquids – blood, phlegm, black bile and yellow bile

INOCULATION putting a low dose of a disease into the body to help it fight against a more serious attack of the same disease

KEYHOLE SURGERY surgical operation performed through a very small incision, using special instruments and an endoscope

LAISSEZ-FAIRE belief that governments should not interfere in people's lives. It prevented public health schemes getting underway in the nineteenth century

LIGATURES a thread used to tie a blood vessel during an operation

'MAGIC BULLETS' pills made from chemicals that kill particular infections inside the body

MEDICAL OFFICER a person appointed to look after the public health of an area

MIASMA smells from decomposing material that were believed to cause disease

MICROBE a tiny single-celled living organism too small to be seen by the naked eye. Disease-causing micro-organisms are called bacteria

MICROSCOPE an instrument that produces magnified images of very small objects

NHS a national health service that is free to everyone and paid for from taxes

NATIONAL INSURANCE gave workers medical help and sick pay if they could not work through illness

PASTEURISATION a process of heating that destroys harmful bacteria

PENICILLIN the first antibiotic drug, produced from the mould penicillium, used to treat infections

PHARMACEUTICAL INDUSTRY large businesses that mass produce drugs for medicine and health care

PHYSICIAN a doctor of medicine who trained at university

PHYSIOLOGY the study of how the body works

PLAGUE a serious infectious disease, bubonic plague was spread to humans by fleas from rats and mice (it first appeared in England as the Black Death in 1348), pneumonic plague spread by people coughing

PUBLIC HEALTH measures taken by the government to look after people's health (acts/laws passed to try and improve public health)

QUACK a person who falsely claims to have medical ability or qualifications

QUININE the drug treatment for malaria

RADIATION THERAPY or radiotherapy, treatment of a disease, such as cancer, by the use of X-rays or similar forms of radiation

REMEDY a drug or treatment that cures or controls the symptoms of a disease

SEWERAGE a system for draining away waste (including human excrement and urine)

SPONTANEOUS GENERATION the theory that decaying matter turns into germs

STAPHYLOCOCCI bacteria found on the skin that can cause infection if the bacteria become trapped

STERILISE to destroy all living micro-organisms from surfaces and surgical instruments, e.g. on a scalpel before an operation

SULPHONAMIDE an antibacterial drug used to treat bronchitis and pneumonia

SUPERBUGS bacteria that have developed immunity to treatment by antibiotics or methods of destroying them by cleaning

SUPERNATURAL something that cannot be given an ordinary explanation

SUPERSTITION an unreasonable belief based on ignorance and sometimes fear

THALIDOMIDE a drug to help morning sickness that was withdrawn in 1961 after it was found to cause limb deformities in babies born to women who had taken it

TRANSFUSION the use of blood given by one person to another when a patient has experienced severe blood loss

TRANSPLANT SURGERY the implanting of tissue or organs from one part of the body to another, or from a donor to a patient

VACCINATION the injection into the body of killed or weakened organisms to give the body resistance against disease

WELFARE STATE a system by which a government takes responsibility for the health and well-being of the population

X-RAYS a photographic or digital image of inside the body

INDEX

acupuncture 77
AIDS (acquired immune deficiency syndrome) 77
air pollution 77
alternative medicine 77, 94
amputation 22, 56–7, 61, 94
amulet 40, 94
anaesthetics 57–9, 80
anatomy 32–3, 94
antibiotic resistance 77
anthrax 53
antibiotics 51, 73–5, 94
antiseptics 60–2, 78, 94
apothecaries 44
artificial limbs 36
arteries 34, 45, 81, 94
Artisan's Dwelling Act 69
aseptic surgery 51, 62, 94
aspirin 76
astrology 14, 15, 27, 94
Bacon, Roger 18
bacteria 50–3, 72
bad air see miasma
barber surgeon 22, 94
Bazalgette, Joseph 69
Bevan, Aneurin 87
Beveridge, William 87
Beveridge Report 87, 94
bezoar stone 39, 94
Black Death 26–7, 94
bleeding, as treatment 15, 38, 94
blood transfusions 78
Booth, Charles 85
Bradmore, John 23
buboes 26, 94
bubonic plague 26, 40–1
burns 79
cancer 80
carbolic acid 60–1, 94
cauterise 22, 37, 94
cesspits 24, 65, 67, 94
Chadwick, Edwin 65–6
Chain, Ernst 74
chemotherapy 80, 94
childbirth 58, 90
children, health of 46–7, 84, 85, 87
chloroform 58–9, 94
cholera 65–7, 94
Christianity, and medicine 12, 18–19
cowpox 46
Crick, Francis 76
Culpepper, Nicholas 38
'cure-alls' 55, 94
Curie, Marie 80
diphtheria 54
diseases
    causes of 14, 19, 40, 50–1, 53, 64
    prevention of 41, 46–7
    treatment of 73–6
dissection 12–13, 16, 30–1, 34, 94
DNA 76, 94
doctors
    Middle Ages 16–18
    Renaissance 44–5

Domagk, Gerhard 55, 73
drinking water 64–5, 67
dysentery 53, 94
Ehrlich, Paul 55, 73
endoscope 81, 95
epidemic 94
ether 57
First World War 72, 79, 86
flagellants 27
Fleming, Alexander 72–3
Florey, Howard 74
Franklin, Rosalind 76
Galen, Claudius 12–13, 16, 18, 32
gangrene 60
genetic illness 76
Germ Theory 50–2, 95
'Great Stink' 64
Gutenberg, Johannes 32
HAART (highly active anti-retroviral therapy) 77
Harvey, William 34
herbal remedies 15, 38, 44, 77, 95
Hill, Octavia 69
Hippocrates 13
home remedies 55
hospitals
    Islamic 20
    Middle Ages 19
    Renaissance 42
    see also surgery
housing 86
Human Genome Project 76
humours 13–15, 95
Hunter, John 45
illness see diseases
immunisation 91
industrialisation 66
    see also nineteenth century
infant mortality 91
infection 22, 59
inoculation 46, 54, 95
Islamic medicine 18, 20–1
Jenner, Edward 45–7
keyhole surgery 81, 95
Koch, Robert 52–3, 73
laughing gas 57
Liberal social reforms 84–5
life expectancy 65, 84, 91
ligatures 37, 95
Lister, Joseph 60–2, 73
Lloyd George, David 85–6
Lower, Richard 45
'magic bullets' 55, 73, 95
magnetic resonance imaging (MRI) 81
measles 54
medicine
    alternative remedies 77, 94
    and Christian Church 12, 18–19
    Galenic 12–13
    herbal remedies 15, 38, 95
    home remedies 55
    Middle Ages 12–16
    nineteenth century 50–5
    pharmaceutical industry 76

quackery 39
Renaissance 30–8, 42–7
twentieth century 72–7, 80–1
see also surgery; vaccinations
mental health 77
miasma 51, 64, 69, 95
Middle Ages
    doctors and physicians 16–18
    hospitals 19
    medicine 12–16, 18
    surgery 22
midwives 17
monasteries 25
Mondeville, Henri de 23
monks 25
National Insurance 85–6, 95
NHS (national health service) 87–90
nineteenth century
    medicine 50–5
    public health 64
    surgery 56–7
nitrous oxide 57
obesity 77
open-heart surgery 81
pain
    as 'good' 59
    during surgery 22, 57
Paré, Ambroise 36–7, 39
Pasteur, Louis 50–1, 54, 69, 73
pasteurisation 50
patent medicines 55
penicillin 72, 74–5, 95
pharmaceutical industry 76, 95
physicians 95
    Middle Ages 16–18
    Renaissance 16–18
    see also doctors; surgeons
physiology 34
plague 15, 26–7, 40–1, 95
plastic surgery 79
pneumonia 55
pneumonic plague 26
polio 54
pollution 77
poverty 65, 84, 86
printing press 32
public health 95
    cesspits 24, 65, 67, 94
    drinking water 64–5, 67
    'Great Stink' 64
    Liberal social reforms 84–5
    life expectancy 65, 84, 91
    sewage 60, 64, 67–9, 95
    see also plague
Public Health Acts 66, 69
purging 38–9
quackery 39, 95
quinine 39, 95
rabies 54
radiation therapy 80, 95
Renaissance
    anatomy, knowledge of 32–3
    medicine 30–8, 42–7
    training and technology 44–5
robotic surgery 81
Rowntree, Seebohm 85

Royal Society 45
scanning machines 81
Second World War 74–5, 87
septicaemia 61
sewage 60, 64, 67–9, 95
Simpson, James 62
smallpox 46–7
Snow, John 67
social reforms 84–5
staphylococcus 73, 95
sterilisation 62, 95
sulphonamide 73, 95
superbugs 77, 95
supernatural 65, 95
superstition 39, 95
surgeons
    barber surgeon 22, 94
    Middle Ages 17, 22–3
    nineteenth century 56–7
    Renaissance 45
surgery
    antiseptic 60–2, 78, 94
    aseptic 51, 62, 94
    development of 82
    and infection 59
    Middle Ages 22–3
    modern methods 80–1
    nineteenth century 56–7
    plastic 79
    Renaissance 36–7
    see also amputation; anaesthetics
syphilis 55
tetanus 54
thalidomide 77, 95
Theory of Opposites 13
Theory of the Four Humours 13, 16, 27
tobacco 39
transfusion see blood transfusions
transplant surgery 81, 95
tuberculosis 52, 54, 55
twentieth century
    housing 86
    medicine 72–7
    surgery 80–1
typhoid 54
unemployment 86
urine chart 15
vaccinations 46–7, 54–5, 73, 95
Vesalius, Andreas 30–3
war and conflict 23, 72, 74–5, 78, 79
waste 15, 24
    see also sewage
Watson, James 76
welfare state 95
Whittington, Richard 19
women
    and childbirth 58, 90
    treating illness 15, 17
    'women searchers' 41
X-rays 78, 81, 95
zodiac chart 15
    see also astrology